Prader–Willi Syndrome

Prader–Willi syndrome (PWS) is associated with an assortment of physical, behavioural and cognitive abnormalities that create a broad range of care needs. Information about the syndrome is spread across a variety of disciplines. In this book the authors seek to identify and provide the latest findings about how best to understand the complex medical, nutritional, psychological, educational, social and therapeutic needs of people with PWS. Their approach is an integrated one, centred on the PWS phenotype. Both authors have been involved in the Cambridge PWS study, which is the largest and most rounded of the cohort studies of PWS anywhere in the world. The unique data it provides are the basis of this book.

Joyce Whittington is a senior research associate and has been instrumental in the running of the Cambridge PWS study.

Tony Holland holds the Chair in Learning Disabilities at Cambridge University and is internationally known in the field of mental retardation.

Prader–Willi Syndrome

Development and Manifestations

Joyce Whittington and Tony Holland

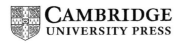

CAMBRIDGE
UNIVERSITY PRESS

PUBLISHED BY THE PRESS SYNDICATE OF THE UNIVERSITY OF CAMBRIDGE
The Pitt Building, Trumpington Street, Cambridge, United Kingdom

CAMBRIDGE UNIVERSITY PRESS
The Edinburgh Building, Cambridge CB2 2RU, UK
40 West 20th Street, New York, NY 10011–4211, USA
477 Williamstown Road, Port Melbourne, VIC 3207, Australia
Ruiz de Alarcón 13, 28014 Madrid, Spain
Dock House, The Waterfront, Cape Town 8001, South Africa

http://www.cambridge.org

First published 2004

Printed in the United Kingdom at the University Press, Cambridge

Typefaces Minion 10.5/14 pt. and Formata   *System* LaTeX 2_ε [TB]

A catalogue record for this book is available from the British Library

Library of Congress Cataloguing in Publication data
Whittington, Joyce.
Prader–Willi Syndrome: development and manifestations / Joyce Whittington, Tony Holland
    p.   cm.
Includes bibliographical references and index.
ISBN 0 521 84029 5 (hardback)
1. Prader–Willi syndrome.   I. Holland, Tony.   II. Prader–Willi Syndrome Association.   III. Title.
RJ520.P7W458   2004   618.92′85884 – dc22   2004040749

ISBN 0 521 84029 5 hardback

Contents

v

Preface

The book follows a process of discovery that included getting to know many people with Prader–Willi syndrome (PWS) and their families through the undertaking of a population-based study of children and adults with PWS living in the then Anglia and Oxford Health Region of the UK. The aims of this study were to systematically investigate many aspects of the syndrome free from the selection biases that may have influenced previous clinic and volunteer-based studies. The in-depth knowledge gained from this 'Cambridge study' through direct contact with people with PWS, their families and other carers, and the integration of this knowledge with that in the literature, has led in turn to new hypotheses and new interpretations of some aspects of PWS.

Prader–Willi syndrome is a relatively rare, genetically determined complex neurodevelopmental disorder. People with the syndrome have their own individual characteristics but share in common particular physical features, specific cognitive strengths and weaknesses, and a propensity to particular behaviours and mental health problems that change with age and together make up the early and later physical and behavioural 'phenotypes' of the syndrome.

The genetics of PWS are still not fully elucidated and are clearly more complex than originally anticipated. Candidate gene(s), located on the long arm of chromosome 15 between bands 11 to 13 (15q11–q13), which are maternally imprinted and only expressed when inherited from the father, have been identified but the precise gene or genes whose absence of expression leads to PWS are still not known.

To understand PWS fully there is the need to integrate research from these diverse fields of genetics and the behavioural, medical and neurosciences. The integration of these scattered and still incomplete areas of knowledge is the central aim of this book. By doing this the pathophysiological mechanisms linking the observed genetic abnormality (genotype) to the physical, behavioural, and psychiatric manifestations (phenotype) of the syndrome can be fully elucidated. This in turn will enable the development of interventions to modify aspects of the phenotype and thereby increase the possibility of a good quality of life for those with the syndrome and their families.

The book is for those who wish to know more about PWS, whether for the purposes of developing research ideas or because he or she is involved in the support of someone with the syndrome. It is written for the professional and the informed reader, and we have attempted to give a comprehensive picture of PWS and thereby of the complex needs of those children and adults with the syndrome. It does not specifically cover those issues directly related to the support of people with the syndrome as these are excellently covered through publications from various national PWS Associations and the International PWS Organisation (PWSA-UK: www.pwsa-uk.demon.co.uk; IPWSO: www.ipwso.org). Books are also available.

The book is centred around 10 research papers (see Appendix P.1) from the Cambridge study that have been published in peer review journals. It also goes well beyond this work. We report on different aspects of our findings and consider the implications of these findings in the context of other published data. Part I describes the characteristics of PWS, the nature of some of the abnormalities of the regulatory mechanisms considered to underpin the phenotypic characteristics, and describes the conception and planning of the Cambridge study. In Part II we systematically consider the findings from the Cambridge study starting with the epidemiological data and then different aspects of the phenotype. In Part III we include other aspects of PWS not considered elsewhere and by the end of the book we have tried to integrate the broad range of observations and to re-conceptualise PWS in a manner that will stimulate thinking and future research.

APPENDIX P.1 PAPERS FROM THE CAMBRIDGE PROJECT

Boer, H., Holland, A. J., Whittington, J. E., Butler, J. V., Webb, T. & Clarke, D. J. Psychotic illness in people with Prader–Willi syndrome due to chromosome 15 maternal uniparental disomy. *Lancet* **359** (2002), 135–136.

Butler, J. V., Whittington, J. E., Holland, A. J., Webb, T., Clarke, D. J. & Boer, H. Prevalence of, and risk factors for, physical ill-health in people with Prader–Willi syndrome: A population-based study. *Developmental Medicine and Child Neurology* **44** (2002), 248–255.

Clarke, D. J., Boer, H., Whittington, J. E., Holland, A. J., Butler, J. V. & Webb, T. Prader–Willi syndrome, compulsive and ritualistic behaviours: the first population-based survey. *British Journal of Psychiatry* **180** (2002), 358–362.

Holland, A. J., Whittington, J. E. & Hinton, E. C. The paradox of Prader–Willi syndrome: a genetic model of starvation. *Lancet* **362** (2003), 989–991.

Holland, A. J., Whittington, J. E., Butler, J., Webb, T., Boer, H. & Clarke, D. Behavioural phenotypes associated with specific genetic disorders: evidence from a population-based study of people with Prader–Willi syndrome. *Psychological Medicine* **33** (2003), 141–153.

Webb, T., Whittington, J., Clarke, D., Boer, H., Butler J. & Holland, A. A study of the influence of different genotypes on the physical and behavioural phenotypes of children and adults ascertained clinically as having PWS. *Clinical Genetics* **62** (2002), 273–281.

Whittington, J. E., Holland, A. J., Webb, T., Butler, J. V., Clarke, D. J. & Boer, H. Population prevalence and estimated birth incidence and mortality rate for people with Prader–Willi syndrome in one UK health region. *Journal of Medical Genetics* **38** (2001), 792–798.

Whittington, J. E., Holland, A. J., Webb, T., Butler, J. V., Clarke, D. J. & Boer, H. Relationship between clinical and genetic diagnosis of Prader–Willi syndrome. *Journal of Medical Genetics* **39** (2002), 926–932.

Whittington, J. E., Holland, A. J., Webb, T., Butler, J. V., Clarke, D. J. & Boer, H. Cognitive abilities and genotype in a population-based sample of people with Prader–Willi syndrome. *Journal of Intellectual Disability Research* **48** (2004), 172–187.

Whittington, J. E., Holland, A. J., Webb, T., Butler, J. V., Clarke, D. J. & Boer, H. Underachievement in Prader–Willi syndrome. *Journal of Intellectual Disability Research* **48** (2004), 188–200.

Acknowledgements

The Cambridge population-based study, which is the focus for this book, was truly a collaborative effort between the Cambridge and Birmingham-based researchers, the UK Prader–Willi Syndrome Association (PWSA), and people with PWS, their families and other carers. We are grateful to all of them and to the Wellcome Trust who were, and continue to be, the main funders of this work. We would also like to thank the UK PWSA and Newton Trust for additional financial support without which this book would not have been possible.

Joyce Whittington and Jill Butler, who undertook the assessments, and Tony Holland are based in the Section of Developmental Psychiatry, Department of Psychiatry, University of Cambridge. Harm Boer and David Clarke are both Consultant Psychiatrists working in the field of learning disability in the NHS in Birmingham in the UK and they took the lead in the mental health and obsessive–compulsive aspects of the study, respectively. Tessa Webb is a Senior Lecturer in the Department of Genetics at the University of Birmingham and undertook the genetic analysis. We would like to acknowledge the essential contributions each have made to the Cambridge study overall and with specific aspects of the study. The respective roles taken by each of the above people are acknowledged through the fact that different people were the lead author for the published papers. In the preparation of this book we are also very grateful to Bonnie Kemske for reading the earlier drafts of each chapter and improving our language and writing style.

People with PWS and their families and other carers willingly contributed to this work and gave up their time to answer many questions and to complete many different assessments. We hope they feel that this book fairly represents, albeit in rather dry and scientific terms, the types of difficulties they experience on a daily basis and that this knowledge will in the end bring about positive changes to their lives.

Part I

Background: Prader–Willi syndrome, why, what, and how to investigate

Background and historical overview

Why study Prader–Willi syndrome?

Prader–Willi Syndrome (PWS) is a genetically determined neurodevelopmental disorder due to one of four presently identified genetic abnormalities that result in the absence of expression of one or more genes at the locus q11–q13 on chromosome 15. Under normal circumstances, these particular genes are expressed when inherited from the father but when of maternal origin they are imprinted (switched off) and therefore in specific tissues are not expressed. The genetic abnormalities associated with PWS result in the alleles of paternal origin being absent and, because the maternal copy is normally imprinted, neither of the alleles of the putative PWS gene(s) are expressed, leading to significant consequences for the developing baby in utero and subsequently throughout the person's lifespan. As described in detail later, PWS is characterised by extreme floppiness (neonatal hypotonia) at birth with failure to thrive and a range of physical, behavioural and cognitive abnormalities that become apparent during development and give rise to often complex health and social needs.

In PWS three significant areas of concern come together. First, there is the developmental delay and the intellectual and functional impairments characteristic of those with an 'intellectual disability'. Second, there is a marked tendency to overeat and the life-threatening obesity that can arise. Third, there is a propensity to particular behaviour patterns and to psychiatric illness that can have a negative impact on the person's quality of life and that of his or her family. Research in these and others areas is required from both theoretical and practical perspectives. With respect to the former, it is necessary to understand the phenomenon, that is, to add to the body of knowledge from a range of perspectives. With respect to the latter, the knowledge gained needs to be used to improve the lives of people with the syndrome, and also to be generalised to similar or related problems, such as obesity, in the general population. The challenge for research is to identify the precise nature of the genetic abnormality (genotype), to identify those physical and behavioural features that are particularly characteristic of the syndrome (phenotype) and to establish the biological and other mechanisms that link genotype to phenotype.

Whilst much has been learnt, the exact nature of the genetic abnormality, and specifically whether one or more genes are involved, is still unknown, as are the underlying brain abnormalities that underpin the behavioural and psychiatric disorders. From the practical perspective, research directed towards identifying and managing the complex medical, nutritional, psychological, educational, social and therapeutic needs of people with PWS is obviously desirable. The fact that many of the physical, cognitive and behavioural manifestations of PWS are present in all, or almost all, people with PWS, and are certainly more prevalent in PWS than in other groups of people with intellectual disabilities, implies a significant involvement of a certain gene or genes located on chromosome 15. The nature and extent of these maladaptive behaviours are likely also to be influenced by factors in the environment and may be ameliorated by suitable interventions. For example, with respect to the physical phenotype, administration of growth hormone from childhood has been shown to have several beneficial effects, as does a controlled diet. Research can contribute to improving the lives of people with PWS through investigating the relative importance of genetic and environmental influences and how then to engineer biological or environmental interventions to bring about beneficial change. In the future, our hope is that research will enable the development of interventions that can significantly reduce some of the most significant physical and behavioural problems associated with the syndrome.

From the point of view of understanding genetic influences on human development, there are features of the syndrome that make it an important field of scientific research. First, the genes, whose absences of expression are thought to be responsible for the syndrome, are imprinted. As PWS is one of the most striking examples of the role of imprinted genes in human development, this discovery has in itself generated a volume of research into imprinted genes, their aetiology and the processes involved. Second, there are two main distinct genotypes for PWS, which lead to subtly different phenotypes. This fact can be exploited so as to localise the genes and eventually the underlying mechanisms responsible for these phenotypic differences, to identify the genes and gene products, and to establish whether they are imprinted or not. Third, there are certain behaviours that are characteristic of all people with the syndrome, that is, common to both the main PWS genotypes, so that PWS is said to have a distinct 'behavioural phenotype'. These observations have only recently begun to be considered in depth, but it is likely that the mechanisms linking individual genes with particular characteristics or behaviours, the associated gene products and their sites of action in the brain will be identified bringing together genetic and behavioural research.

The scientific questions to which answers are sought include: the identities of the PWS gene(s) and the gene products, the normal sites of expression of the genes and their modes of action particularly in the brain, the identities of the genes that are presumed to be responsible for differences between the genetic subtypes; and, from a clinical perspective, why some physical and behavioural characteristics are invariably present and others are not, and what are the underlying causative mechanisms? Possible hypothetical models linking genotype to phenotype and how such hypothetical models might be tested are considered in Chapter 8.

Historical perspective of PWS

People with PWS have no doubt been born throughout history (the 6-year-old girl, Eugenia Martinez Vallejo, whose pictures, painted by Juan Carreno de Miranda in about 1680 are in the Prado museum may well have PWS), but because of the neonatal hypotonia and feeding difficulties common to babies with PWS, few such infants may have survived prior to the advent of better neonatal care. The second, over-eating (hyperphagic) phase, which begins after weaning, would therefore have been rarely observed in those days and then only in isolated individuals. The advent of improved mother and baby care, especially of feeding techniques (such as tube feeding), made it possible for significant numbers of babies with the syndrome to survive and, hence, groups of people with apparent similar characteristics to be noticed and eventually reported in the scientific literature. Such reports describing the characteristics of a small number of people with an apparent syndrome led in turn to further reports and ultimately to more systematic investigation.

In 1956,[1] the Swiss paediatricians Prader, Labhart and Willi first described a group of children with what subsequently came to be called PWS. The main features noted at that time were neonatal hypotonia, impaired sexual development, short stature, a propensity to severe obesity, and learning disabilities (mental retardation). In 1963, Prader and Willi[2] reported 14 Swiss children with similar characteristics, as did Laurance[3] in England who described six children. Reports also followed from other parts of the world, from: Canada (Dunn *et al.*, 1961)[4]; France (Gabilan, 1962)[5]; United States (Zellweger *et al.*, 1962)[6]; Spain (Sanchez Villares *et al.*, 1964)[7]; Sweden (Forssman & Hagberg, 1964)[8]; Netherlands (Monnens & Kenis, 1965)[9]; and Belgium (Hooft *et al.*, 1966)[10]. In a later paper describing nine children, together with a review of other papers, Laurance listed the main features as: neuromuscular (neonatal hypotonia), 'mental disorders' (i.e. IQs in the lowest 2% of the population), abnormalities in body configuration (obesity and poor growth), skeletal disorders (mainly scoliosis), characteristic facial appearance (almond-shaped eyes, high cranial vault), endocrine abnormalities (risk of diabetes mellitus) and delayed gonadal development.[11] Other features now recognised as being common, for example, an apparently high pain threshold, were also noted.

As more people were identified with the syndrome, advances were made in delineating common characteristics and in distinguishing PWS from other conditions with some similar features. Zellweger and Schneider[12] described 14 people with the syndrome and reviewed the literature on 79 others. They distinguished the early hypotonic stage of feeding difficulties from the obese, food obsessed second stage. They also reported non-consistency of some of the abnormalities that had been reported associated with the syndrome (for example, diabetes mellitus and daytime sleepiness). Hall & Smith[13] tabulated the abnormalities that were found to affect 32 people with PWS. It is of note that they found hypotonia, feeding problems, delayed developmental milestones, male hypogenitalism and obesity in 100% of those they considered to have PWS. Decreased fetal movements, 'mental deficiency' (low IQ), 'personality problems', short stature, delayed bone age, acromicria (small hands and feet) and male cryptorchidism (undescended testes) were found in over half of those with PWS described. This article also drew attention to the temper tantrums and stubbornness that often occur from childhood and reported that by late adolescence and adulthood almost all of the individuals had serious 'personality problems'.

One of the most prominent features of PWS is the abnormal interest in food, the eating behaviour (hyperphagia), and the resultant obesity. In the early years most of the people diagnosed following the identification of the syndrome were already well into the second phase and severely obese. When a young child was diagnosed with PWS, while still in the first phase of the syndrome, his growth was monitored into the second phase. His weight began to increase out of proportion to height and efforts were made to restrict his eating by means of a diet designed for children of that age and build. It was found that such a diet still resulted in rapid weight increase, showing that the caloric requirements of people with PWS were less than expected.[14] For some years now, detailed dietary advice and advice on food management has been available to parents and carers of people diagnosed with PWS in many countries but, if the diagnosis of PWS was made later in life after the onset of obesity, it was too late to avoid the formation of problematic eating habits and associated medical problems. Given the problems of over-eating and the need to prevent obesity it is now recognised that early diagnosis is particularly important.

Impact of PWS clinics

The complexity of needs of people with PWS led to the recognition that the skills of different professionals were required: dieticians, paediatricians, psychiatrists, and psychologists to help advise on the prevention of obesity and on the other behaviours; occupational and physical therapists for the hypotonia and inactivity; speech and language therapists for speech problems; educational psychologists and educators to assess and ameliorate the consequences of developmental delay and learning disabilities; and family support services for parents. For this reason the first PWS clinic was established in the United States in 1972 at the University of Washington, with professionals available to cover the above areas of need; others subsequently followed.

The results of such clinics were, first, that problems could be recognised early and dealt with immediately. Second, parents were able to meet others facing the same kinds of difficulties, and could exchange experiences and support one another. Third, it enabled research to be undertaken based on people with PWS seen in these clinics. Such research had its strengths and weaknesses. One major concern was the absence at that time of agreed diagnostic criteria and no genetic test was then available. In the absence of established and valid criteria and a sound genetic test, diagnosis was potentially problematic, only improving with the development of proper diagnostic criteria and ultimately the identification of the genetic abnormality.

Impact of PWS associations

The success of PWS clinics in bringing families of people with PWS together and the formation of local groups of such families, along with the growing perception of the need for support and information services, led to the formation of national PWS associations. The first of these was American in 1975, followed by the UK Association in 1981. In 1991 the International Prader–Willi Syndrome Organisation (IPSWO) was established bringing together over 30 national associations. These associations have had important impacts on knowledge about, and support for, people with PWS. They were (and still are) the first resource for most families with a newly diagnosed baby with PWS. The associations provide emotional and practical support when crises arise and information about the syndrome when needed. Whilst those who are directly concerned with the support of a person with PWS may become knowledgeable, local medical, social and educational services tended to remain in ignorance, and even today one can still find attitudes that reflect this ignorance. For example, we found that one local authority agreed to pay for a man with PWS to go to a PWS home for a limited period of six months so that he could 'lose a bit of weight and sort himself out'; and another thought that 'all learning disabled people are alike, we do not distinguish people with PWS from the rest'. The second impact of the establishment of associations has been on research. Access to an association mailing list has meant that larger groups of people with

PWS could be contacted for questionnaire and other studies. Although this means of ascertainment raises concern about potential bias, the larger numbers have given more statistical power to the analyses of the data collected.

In 1977, researchers from the Washington PWS clinic undertook a questionnaire survey of parents and professionals who had written to the clinic about the syndrome. Returned questionnaires identified 98 people, out of 106 returns, diagnosed with PWS by other physicians, who also satisfied the clinic's own criteria. These, together with reports in the literature and opinions of physicians attending a PWS Workshop at the University of Washington in 1979, formed the basis of the first set of Consensus Diagnostic Criteria.[15] At that time it was agreed that symptoms essential for diagnosis included: infantile central hypotonia; hypogonadism; obesity; cognitive and learning disabilities; short stature for familial background; and dysmorphic facial features. Infantile central hypotonia is often associated with abnormal delivery and almost always associated with poor suck, feeding problems, and delayed motor landmarks. Hypogonadism, or abnormal development of physical sexual characteristics, is difficult to diagnose in infancy in females but less so in males, since undescended testes are common. Later it is often manifested in absent or infrequent menstrual periods in adult females and a small penis in adult males. Following the failure to thrive in infancy, obesity can occur in the absence of intervention to limit access to food. When food intake is controlled, the propensity to obesity is still apparent, in that the person's caloric requirement is low and the distribution of subcutaneous fat tissue is more prolific on the lower trunk, buttocks, and thighs. The cognitive and learning disabilities in PWS are not always associated with a low IQ, but educational attainment, relative to measured IQ, is generally disappointing, with arithmetic being worse than reading. Short-term memory and comprehension of abstract concepts are usually weak compared to visuo-spatial skills. Although most people with PWS are short, some people with PWS are above the 10th centile for height, these tend to be those with very tall parents, for whom one would predict a height above the 95th centile. Such people are therefore of short stature for familial background. Dysmorphic facial features, associated with PWS, include a high narrow forehead, almond-shaped eyes, and a triangular mouth, but these are not so pronounced when obesity is prevented.

All other symptoms reported to occur in people with PWS were not consistently present, each reportedly occurring in less than 100% of those with the syndrome. The prevalence of these symptoms in the questionnaire survey could be affected by response bias and might not be representative of the total PWS population. However, based on this survey, the desirability of the adoption of diagnostic criteria for PWS was first recognised, in order to improve the ability of clinicians to accurately diagnose the syndrome.

Consensus Diagnostic Criteria (CDC)

Ten years after the first proposal for the adoption of diagnostic criteria for PWS, the need for clinical diagnostic criteria was seen to be threefold: (a) for use by practicing clinicians in diagnosis; (b) as a screening instrument to identify the advisability of genetic testing, ideally in early childhood; and (c) to ensure more uniformity and reliability in those taking part in research studies. Seven professionals, each with many years of clinical experience with PWS, developed lists of diagnostic criteria for PWS. These were then assessed by five of these professionals on 113 people previously diagnosed with PWS. Minor alterations were made in the criteria following discussion at several scientific meetings. The final criteria were published as the Consensus Diagnostic Criteria in 1993.[16] They were divided into three groups: eight major criteria; eleven minor criteria; and eight supportive findings. Major criteria scored one point, minor criteria scored half a point and supportive findings were not scored but were said to increase the certainty of diagnosis. The two distinct phases of PWS were acknowledged, in that the requirements for diagnosis were distinct for ages 0–3 years (five or more points at least four of which are major) and 3 years to adulthood (eight or more points at least five of which are major). It is to be noted that no specific criterion was required to be present, merely that the total numbers present reached the minimum specified. The relationship between these criteria and PWS genetics will be considered further in Chapter 5.

Prevalence of PWS

The physicians consulted in the first Consensus Diagnostic Criteria debate also reached agreement on the birth incidence of PWS as roughly 1:10 000. Other estimates followed, mainly based on surveys of physicians with experience of diagnosing PWS, and the agreed prevalence was generally quoted as between 1:15 000 and 1:25 000. Prior to our Cambridge study, only two estimates appear to be based on epidemiological data, those of Akefeldt *et al.*, published in 1991,[17] and Burd *et al.*, published in 1990.[18] In the latter North Dakota study, the authors surveyed paediatricians, neurologists, and clinical geneticists, and also contacted the state's comprehensive evaluation centre, the state hospital, the state institution for the 'mentally retarded', and group homes for the developmentally disabled, including one for people with PWS. In most communities, at least four of these sources of information were consulted. Each was sent a one-page questionnaire pictorially demonstrating the signs of PWS to aid identification. The response rate was 99%. These procedures resulted in the identification of eight males, eight females, and one person whose gender was not given, with an age range from 9 to 30 years.

At that time the population of North Dakota for that age range was 263 444, giving a prevalence rate of 1:16 062, equivalent to 1:38 395 in the entire population. No figures were given for the number of people with an established genetic diagnosis.

In the Akefeldt study, the authors estimated the prevalence of PWS in the age range 0 to 25 years in the rural Swedish county of Skaraborg, by surveying paediatricians, neuropaediatricians, child psychiatrists, school health visitors, general practitioners and doctors working in the fields of general medicine, rehabilitation and mental disabilities. The authors circulated diagnostic criteria for PWS to these professionals and also invited all school nurses in the county to seminars where the features of PWS were described. Requests were made that they should be informed about all people with possible PWS. All people with possible PWS were examined by a neuropaediatrician, a child psychiatrist, a child psychologist and a speech pathologist. Clinical diagnoses were made on the basis of their findings. Eleven people (seven male and four female) were considered to definitely have PWS and a further five (two male and three female) were considered probable. These numbers gave a population prevalence of 'clear PWS' up to age 25 years of 1:8500 and between 7 to 25 years, 1:8000. If the people with suspected PWS were also included, these prevalence rates became 1: 6700 and 1:5000, respectively. As discussed in a later chapter, it is likely that these were significant over-estimates of the prevalence rates.

Mortality in PWS

The North Dakota study, mentioned above, found no people with PWS over the age of 30. In the PWS literature, very few older people have been described with genetically confirmed PWS. An exception is the report[19] of a woman who died aged 71 years, who was found to have a chromosomal deletion characteristic of PWS. There is a report of two older women (aged 54 and 69) in 1988,[20] but the diagnoses had only been made on clinical grounds. The Cambridge study found several older adults who may have PWS on clinical grounds, but all those genetically tested over the age of 47 years were subsequently found not to have the PWS genotype. The observation of an apparent lack of older people with the syndrome suggests that there is a significant mortality rate in later life, but such studies cannot rule out the unlikely possibility that older people with PWS are living in the community but have never been recognised as having the syndrome.

Anecdotally, the probable increased mortality of older people with PWS has been attributed to obesity-related deaths that have been thought to be most prevalent in early adulthood, when parental control over access to food has had to be relaxed or relinquished. More recently, this latter view has been challenged. At the 2001 International PWS Organisation conference, one speaker described sudden deaths in PWS occurring at all ages. Moreover, findings from our study were interpreted as showing a linear increased mortality rate across the age range (not just in later life) compared to the general population (see Chapter 4).

Genetics of PWS

Normally a person has 23 pairs of chromosomes, one of each pair being inherited from the mother and one from the father. One of the 23 pairs make up the sex chromosomes (XY in males and XX in females). The other 22 are referred to as the autosomes. When scientific and technical progress made it possible to see chromosomes under a microscope, distinct pairs were identified and numbered in decreasing order of size from 1 to 22, and on other characteristics (position of the centromere and the banding pattern on staining) as chromosomal staining became more sophisticated. It was also realised that structural abnormalities of various kinds could affect the chromosomes and many of these abnormalities were subsequently shown to be associated with abnormal mental and/or physical development, depending on the particular chromosomal defect and on the particular chromosome(s) involved.

From the late 1970s, occasional reports appeared in the literature suggesting that PWS was associated with a deletion or a translocation (chromosomal re-arrangment) affecting a certain part of one of the pair of chromosome 15s. Less than a decade later, it was estimated that in 50% of people with PWS there was a small deletion of a certain part of the long arm of one of the chromosome 15s, now called the PWS critical region and denoted by the term 15q11–q13, indicating that the deletion is between bands 11 and 13. Chromosomal re-arrangments, such as translocations, made up less than 5% and included most of the people with familial PWS, with the chromosomal translocation being inherited from the father. More recent research has shown that the DNA of the PWS region is bounded by unstable DNA repeat sequences,[21] so that breakage at these boundaries is more likely than in stable regions lacking such repeats, thus explaining why such structural chromosomal abnormalities occur involving the chromosomal region 15q11–q13.

Observation that a deletion of the same small region of one of the chromosome 15s could lead to a totally different syndrome – Angelman syndrome – together with the advent of molecular genetics (which does not rely on direct visual examination of chromosome areas), led to two new discoveries relating to the genetics of PWS. First, the particular chromosome 15 associated with a deletion resulting in PWS was that copy inherited from the father. A deletion of a similar area of the chromosome 15 inherited from the mother resulted in Angelman syndrome. Second, in most cases of PWS that were not associated with a deletion of the PWS region, another chromosomal abnormality existed in which both copies of chromosome 15 had been inherited from the mother (there was no paternal copy). These were called maternal disomies and, more specifically, heterodisomy when the maternal copies were distinct and isodisomy when the same maternal copy was duplicated. The process responsible for disomy is hypothesised to be 'trisomy rescue'. Trisomies, three copies of a given chromosome, are fairly common genetic faults that result from non-disjunction of chromosomes during cell division. Many trisomies are non-viable and result in spontaneous abortions or in early postnatal death. If one of the three chromosome copies can be rejected by the early dividing cell, the fetus can be 'rescued' and will be viable in this situation. Inheriting both copies of one pair of chromosomes from one parent is problematic when one or more of the several thousand genes on a chromosome is imprinted. Under these circumstances, whether a gene is switched on or off will depend on the gender of the parent from whom the gene is inherited. If there are no imprinted genes on the chromosome, then it is likely that the fetus will be normal. However, in the case of chromosome 15, retention of two copies from the mother results in PWS, while retention of two copies from the father results in Angelman syndrome. It was the observations that only deletion of q11–q13 on a chromosome 15 of paternal origin and only maternal disomy 15 resulted in PWS (as opposed to maternal deletion or paternal disomy) that were the important clues that the PWS gene or genes must be imprinted (switched off) when inherited from the mother and normally expressed when inherited from the father (see Figure 1.1).

PWS genes are maternally imprinted and normally only the copy inherited from the father is active. Since this copy is missing in PWS due to a chromosomal deletion and both copies are imprinted in those with the maternal disomy, the normal gene actions are absent, resulting in the characteristic manifestations of the syndrome. In the case of Angelman syndrome, about 20% of people with the syndrome have a mutation of a single gene, UBE3A. These include most of the familial cases. In contrast, in PWS familial cases are rare, either associated with an imprinting centre fault or with unbalanced translocations involving breakage points in the 15q11–q13 region. No single gene has yet been found to be causally associated with PWS. Although SNRPN is the strongest candidate gene, PWS is still generally considered to be a polygenic disorder, the result of the non-functioning of several genes. More recently, on the basis of behavioural data, we have challenged this view.[22] The 15q11–q13 region is still poorly defined, with few paternally expressed genes having been identified and, to date, no single mutation in any of them (other than the imprinting centre) has definitively been associated with any clinical signs or symptoms. The most common cause of PWS is a 4 megabase (Mb) deletion and attempts to find a common region of overlap among those with deletions in PWS have only reduced the size of the necessary chromosomal deletion to about half.

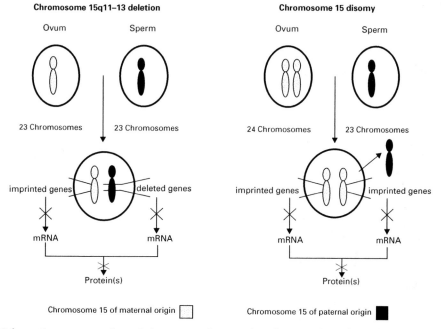

Figure 1.1.   Schematic representation of the two main genetic subtypes of Prader–Willi syndrome (PWS).

Imprinting in both PWS and Angelman syndrome is controlled by an imprinting centre in the PWS region of chromosome 15 (15q11–q13). Current research centres on delineating the various areas within the imprinting centre and the extent to which this imprinting centre influences nearby genes, the degree of effectiveness of imprinting, and the mechanisms by which imprinting is achieved. Abnormalities in what is described as 'an imprinting centre' or the imprinting process have been found to lead to PWS and are also responsible for some very rare familial cases of PWS.[23] The imprinting centre covers about 100 kilobase (kb) of genomic sequence but is bipartite in structure, as deletions of the proximal portion result in Angelman syndrome, while deletions of the distal portion of the imprinting centre are associated with PWS. The PWS imprinting control element spans the promotor and exon 1 of the *SNRPN* gene. The shortest region of overlap observed in imprinting centre mutations has established its size as about 4.3 kb. The PWS element switches the grandmaternal imprint to a paternal epigenotype in the father. One of the mechanisms governing the establishment of this parent-of-origin epigenetic modification is methylation of specific DNA sequences. This has been exploited in the molecular diagnosis of PWS.

The advent of a genetic test that can detect almost all people with PWS, by considering the methylation status at *SNRPN*, is a landmark in PWS research. It is now possible to ensure that participants in PWS research groups are all genetically confirmed. Moreover, all previous reported results, based on a mixture of genetically and clinically diagnosed participants, can be re-assessed by repeating those studies using only those participants with a genetic diagnosis. In the following chapters, priority will be given to research using participants with genetically confirmed PWS, in preference to those clinically diagnosed, or mixed groups. The reality of having PWS for the individual concerned still remains difficult but the possibility of early diagnosis has helped to bring interventions that, whilst not directly solving the fundamental problems, can prevent obesity and help to improve some physical aspects through the use of growth hormone. In the subsequent chapters we consider in greater detail different aspects of PWS, drawing specifically on the findings from our Cambridge population-based study.

Summary

Prader–Willi syndrome is generally a non-heritable genetically determined condition.

Behaviourally, there are two distinct phases: hypotonic, failure to thrive babies; and hyperphagic children and adults with behavioural and psychiatric problems.

Genetically, there are two main genotypes which have few, but very important differences.

REFERENCES

1. Prader, A., Labhart, A. & Willi, H. Ein Syndrom von Adipositas, Kleinwuchs, Kryptorchismus und Oligophrenie nach myatonieartigem Zustand in Neugeborenenalter. *Schweizerische Medizinische Wochenschrift* **86** (1956), 1260–1261.

2. Prader, A. & Willi, H. Das Syndrom von Imbezillitat, Adipositas, Muskelhypotonie, Hypogenitalismus, Hypogonadismus und Diabetes mellitus mit 'Myatonie' -Anamnese. *Second International Congress on Mental Retardation, Vienna, 1961*, p. 353. Basel: S. Karger, 1963.

3. Laurance, B. M. The first four cases of reference 11, reported at the *32nd Annual Meeting of the British Paediatric Association in Cambridge*, 1961.

4. Dunn, H. G., Ford, D. K., Auersperg, N. & Miller, J. R. Benign congenital hypotonia with chromosomal anomaly. *Pediatrics* **28** (1961), 578–591.

5. Gabilan, J. C. Syndrome de Prader, Labhart et Willi. *Journal de Pediat* **1** (1962), 179.

6. Zellweger, H. U., Smith, J. W. & Cusminsky, M. Muscular hypotonia in infancy: diagnosis and differentiation. *Revue Canadienne de Biologie* **21** (1962), 599–612.

7. Sanchez Villares, E., Martin Esteban, M. & Durantez Mayo, O. Amiotonia congenita con sindrome de Prader–Willi incompleto. *Boletin de la Sociedad Castellano-Astur-Leonesa de Pediatria* **5** (1964), 191–208.

8. Forssman, H. & Hagberg, B. Prader–Willi syndrome in boy of ten with prediabetes. *Acta Paediatrica* **53** (1964), 70–78.

9. Monnens, L. & Kenis, H. Enkele onderzoekingen bij een patient met het syndroom van Prader–Willi. *Maandschrift vor Kindergeneeskunde* **33** (1965), 482–498.

10. Hooft, C., Delire, C. & Casneuf, J. Le syndrome de Prader–Labhardt–Willi–Fanconi: Etude clinique, endocrinologique et cytogenetique. *Acta Paediatrica Belgica* **20** (1966), 27–50.

11. Laurance, B. M. Hypotonia, mental retardation, obesity, and cryptorchidism associated with dwarfism and diabetes in children. *Archives of Disease in Childhood* **42** (1967), 126–139.

12. Zellweger, H. & Schneider, H. J. Syndrome of hypotonia–hypomentia–hypogonadism–obesity (HHHO) or Prader–Willi syndrome. *American Journal of Diseases of Children* **115** (1968), 588–598.

13. Hall, B. D. & Smith, D. W. Prader–Willi syndrome. A resume of 32 cases including an instance of affected first cousins, one of whom is of normal stature and intelligence. *Pediatrics* **81** (1972), 286–293.

14. Pipes P. L. & Holm, V. A. Weight control of children with Prader–Willi syndrome. *Journal of the American Dietetic Association* **62** (1973), 520–524.

15. Holm, V. A. The diagnosis of Prader–Willi syndrome. In Holm, V. A., Sulzbacher, S. & Pipes, P. L. (Eds). *The Prader–Willi Syndrome*, pp. 27–44. Baltimore: University Park Press, 1981.

16. Holm, V. A., Cassidy S. B., Butler, M. G. *et al.* Prader–Willi syndrome: Consensus Diagnostic Criteria. *Pediatrics* **91** (1993), 398–402.

17. Akefeldt, A., Gillberg, C. & Larsson, C. Prader–Willi syndrome in a Swedish rural county: epidemiological aspects. *Developmental Medicine and Child Neurology* **33** (1991), 715–721.

18. Burd, L., Vesely, B., Martsolf, J. & Kerbeshian, J. Prevalence study of Prader–Willi syndrome in North Dakota. *American Journal of Medical Genetics* **37** (1990), 97–99.

19. Carpenter, P. K. Prader–Willi syndrome in old age. *Journal of Intellectual Disability Research* **38** (1994), 529–531.

20. Goldman, J. J. Prader–Willi syndrome in two institutionalised older adults. *Mental Retardation* **26** (1988), 97–102.

21. Amos-Landgraf, J. M., Ji, Y., Gottlieb, W. *et al.* Chromosome breakage in the Prader–Willi and Angelman syndromes involves recombination between large, transcribed repeats at proximal and distal breakpoints. *American Journal of Human Genetics* **65** (1999), 370–386.

22. Holland, A. J., Whittington, J. E. & Hinton, E. C. The paradox of Prader–Willi syndrome: a genetic model of starvation. *Lancet* **362** (2003), 989–991.

23. Buiting, K., Dittrich, B., Gross, S. *et al.* Sporadic imprinting defects in Prader–Willi syndrome and Angelman syndrome: implications for imprint-switch models, genetic counseling, and prenatal diagnosis *American Journal of Human Genetics* **63** (1998), 170–180.

2

Biological and regulatory mechanisms in PWS

The areas of research considered in this chapter were not directly included in the Cambridge population-based study. However, these studies are important in that they further identified some of the possible pathophysiological mechanisms that underpin the physical and behavioural characteristics that the diagnostic criteria have identified as being central to the syndrome. For example, the very striking features of obesity, short stature and impaired sexual development, together with the less obvious features of temperature dysregulation, abnormal pain threshold and abnormal body composition, all require an explanation. In essence, it is important to establish whether these apparently diverse abnormalities might be traced back to a common single causal mechanism (and by implication the absence of expression of one gene) and, if so, whether the fundamental biological deficits consequent upon the PWS genotype are central (i.e. an abnormality of brain function) or more peripheral and due to abnormal feedback mechanisms, for example, from the gut and/or fat stores. An alternative view is that PWS should be seen as a 'contiguous gene disorder' and that it is the absence of expression of more than one imprinted gene that leads to the full PWS phenotype. If more than one gene is involved, then there may not be a single unifying pathophysiology, but rather, different and discrete pathological mechanisms that lead to particular phenotypic abnormalities.

One key aim of the Cambridge population-based study was to address this fundamental question of whether all that is observed in PWS can be accounted for by one mechanism or whether more than one discrete mechanism is involved and by implication more than one gene. To address this issue, a detailed description of the PWS phenotype, the relationship with age, and the extent to which particular behavioural characteristics are always present or only sometimes present is crucial. We review these studies early in the book, as they informed our thinking when designing the investigations that made up the Cambridge population-based study.

Most of the findings described in this and later chapters are based on our studies of children and adults with PWS. However, methods are also needed that enable the investigation of putative neurobiological abnormalities that may account for some of the behavioural and cognitive characteristic of those with PWS. Such investigations have included the study of brain tissue obtained, with consent, after death from people with PWS and the development of animal models. These two research strategies enable the investigation into the fundamental consequences of the PWS genetic abnormality and putative brain mechanisms that mediate between the genotype and the phenotype. In particular, since genes are often only expressed in certain organs, or only in certain cells, it is important to know in which tissues, and specifically which areas of the brain, the imprinted 'PWS gene(s)' are normally expressed and are functional, and therefore by implication not able to be expressed or functional in those with PWS. This differential gene expression means that studying gene expression in humans from the white blood cells of blood alone is unlikely to be informative about other tissues.

In the case of PWS, the study of animals and the creation of 'animal models' of PWS have been useful in two broad ways, particularly with respect to understanding the basis of the abnormal eating behaviour. First, studies involving the manipulation of certain brain areas and nuclei have been crucially important[1,2] in the identification of the nuclei in the hypothalamus of the brain whose actions increase or decrease feeding behaviour. For example, it has been known for many years that lesions of different areas within the hypothalamus result, respectively, in hyperphagia and obesity and in food avoidance and starvation. These early observations gave rise to the idea of 'hunger' and 'satiety' centres. This model is now more commonly thought of as collections of neurones whose synapses express specific neurotransmitters that mediate effects on food intake and/or energy expenditure, regulated by signals of nutritional state.[3] The control of eating behaviour would appear to be mediated centrally by the hypothalamus and peripherally by feedback from the gut and fat tissue to the hypothalamus via the vagus nerve or by the effects of hormones such as leptin, ghrelin and cholecystokinin.[4] This process is referred to as the 'satiety cascade.[5] The task in PWS research is to tease out the relative importance of the different parts of these peripheral and central feedback mechanisms to further our understanding of the eating behaviour.

Second, mouse animal models, in which genetic abnormalities similar to those in PWS have been created in laboratory mice, allow the study of underlying brain abnormalities and the links between specific genetic lesions and abnormal behaviour. From a genetic perspective, the mouse chromosome 7 is very similar to the human chromosome 15. In addition, many brain areas have similar functions in all mammals. While there are obvious limitations when drawing inferences about humans from the study of such animals, such methods provide the means for investigating gene expression and neurotransmitter activity in ways that would not be possible in humans. Whilst the diversity of the PWS phenotype indicates that different neural systems are affected, much of what is observed in PWS indicates that there is a disorder of regulatory mechanisms controlled through the counterbalancing actions of different hypothalamic nuclei. Thus, crucial to the understanding of the PWS phenotype is the investigation of the brain nuclei that make up the hypothalamus and the feedback mechanisms that influence hypothalamic function.

The role of the hypothalamus

Findings from previous studies indicate that the regulation of systems controlling growth, sexual development and eating behaviour are abnormal in all those with PWS, while those systems controlling birth processes, sleep, temperature and pain are abnormal in many with PWS but not all (see Chapter 1). All of these systems are regulated partially or wholly within the hypothalamus and it is generally agreed that some hypothalamic abnormality underlies the PWS phenotype.[6] These abnormalities are summarised below.

Pregnancy, fetal function, birth and the neonatal stage

One of the best-documented features of PWS is the severe hypotonia at birth that may persist into childhood. Hypotonia has been suggested as the cause for decreased fetal movements during pregnancy, for abnormal presentation at birth, and for long labour, all of which are often observed in the case of babies born with PWS.[6] Gestation may be abnormally short or long and the percentage of babies suffering from asphyxia has been reported to be much higher than in the general population.[7] In the Cambridge study, decreased fetal movements were reported in 76% of those mothers of children with PWS interviewed (Chapter 5), and some abnormality of pregnancy or birth was reported in 66%, including breech birth in 19%, and abnormally long labour in over 7%. Almost 25% were a month or more premature, while almost 20% were two or more weeks late. To the extent that known hypothalamic damage, such as that from anencephaly and septo-optic dysplasia, results in similar abnormalities of presentation, long labour and premature or postmature birth in the absence of hypotonia, the hypothalamus has been implicated in the aetiology of these particular characteristics.[8,9]

Sex hormones and fertility in PWS

Undersized sex organs in those of either gender, decreased sexual behaviour and the absence of the normal growth spurt, as well as undescended testes in boys and delayed or absent menarche in girls are characteristic of PWS (Chapters 5 and 9). These abnormalities are thought to be wholly or partly the results of decreased levels of sex hormones in children with PWS arising from abnormal function of hypothalamic luteinising hormone-releasing hormone neurones.[6]

It was thought that, as a result of these hormonal abnormalities, people with PWS were infertile, but in the past decade there have been two reports of women with PWS who have given birth. One mother had PWS due to a deletion involving the PWS chromosomal region. As the genetic understanding of PWS and Angelman syndrome would predict, she had a 50% chance of giving birth to a child with Angelman syndrome. This was in fact what happened.[10] The other mother had PWS due to maternal disomy and gave birth to a normal baby.[11] No example of male fertility has yet been described in the literature. In one study, testosterone levels in a group of men with PWS[12] were reduced in most of them, but not all.

Obesity, growth and body composition in PWS

Perhaps the most characteristic feature of PWS is the over-eating behaviour, which, in the absence of intervention, inevitably leads to severe obesity. Since the resulting obesity is highly likely to lead to serious medical conditions and possibly early death (see Chapter 9), it is a major cause for concern. Moreover, it is exacerbated by the short stature of most people with the syndrome. Whilst subsequent studies (reviewed below) have changed the emphasis from seeing PWS as a syndrome of obesity to a syndrome of abnormal and excessive eating behaviour, it is now clearly established that the abnormal body composition and associated reduced energy-use contribute to the physical appearance and to the difficulty experienced by people with PWS in preventing obesity.

The short stature of people with PWS has been attributed primarily to the decreased levels of growth hormone. The short stature appears to be present from birth (birth length in PWS has been reported to be less than normal[13]) and this is compounded by a lack of growth spurt prior to the time puberty would normally occur.[14] It has long been known that growth hormone levels are low in people with PWS and a study published in 1998[15] concluded that this was a cause of the short stature and that impaired growth hormone secretion is not secondary to obesity. A considerable amount of research has been directed to studies of the effects of growth hormone treatment. These have confirmed that it is the primary low level of growth hormone and not the inability to utilise it that accounts for some of the abnormalities in growth and body composition in PWS.[16,17,18,19] These studies have also demonstrated the role of growth hormone deficiency in some of the physical features of PWS; for example, hands and feet have grown disproportionately and facial features have been considered to change[19] after growth hormone replacement. It is generally agreed that the effects of growth hormone treatment on PWS children, in variable doses[16,17,18,19] and for periods of six months to one year or more, include: increased growth velocity; decreased percentage body fat and increased percentage lean mass; improved respiratory muscle function, and increased physical strength and agility; and decreased skinfold thickness. Most studies have found no significant change in body weight compared with an untreated comparison group with PWS. It is now thought that the changes in body composition and activity level are even more beneficial than the height gain, and research in this area has been directed towards possible beneficial effects of growth hormone treatment in adults and babies, rather than just during childhood. In spite of earlier fears about possible exacerbation of scoliosis as a result of growth hormone treatment, in practice very few such effects have been reported.

Body composition in PWS has been shown to be atypical compared to other forms of obesity. People with PWS have been compared with similarly obese people without PWS and, in some studies, with a matched normal weight group.[20,21,22,23,24] One comprehensive study[24] compared total body analysis of 27 people aged 6 to 22 years with PWS with that of an obese comparison group matched on age, gender and BMI, and with that of a non-obese comparison group matched on age and gender. Total percentage body fat was significantly greater in PWS than in the obese group; a similar difference was found for arms and legs but not for trunk. Lean mass was significantly lower in PWS than in both comparison groups and the most affected regions were the limbs, so that the ratio of lean mass in the trunk to that in the limbs was significantly higher in PWS than in the two comparison groups. The ratio of fat mass to lean mass was significantly higher in those with PWS than in those in the obese comparison group.

Bone mineral content was significantly lower in those with PWS than in the other two groups. This was especially true in the limbs. Bone mineral density in PWS was similar to that in the normal comparison group but significantly lower than that in the obese comparison group. Comparing two age subgroups (<12years, ≥12years) of the PWS group, the study found that older people with PWS had higher adiposity, lower bone mineral content and dramatically lower bone mineral density. One paper looked at younger children with PWS before the onset of obesity[25] and found elevated skinfold thickness and elevated leptin levels, relative to prediction based on BMI, in these underweight (for height) PWS infants. The authors concluded that body composition is abnormal before the onset of obesity. The body composition has a particular influence on energy expenditure, which is low in PWS.[20,21,23] These referenced studies suggest that the low energy expenditure is due to the small lean mass in PWS and not to any difference in efficiency at the cellular level.

The eating disturbance in PWS

Abnormal and excessive eating behaviour is universal in children and adults with PWS, and if not present suggests an incorrect diagnosis. However, there is some variation in the nature and severity of this behaviour (see Chapter 5). Strikingly, this propensity to excessive eating behaviour is not present from birth. Babies with PWS are initially hypotonic, and have a poor suck, usually necessitating tube feeding, and in early infancy they fail to thrive. At this stage of development they appear to have no interest in feeding. At some point, usually in the first two years, appetite appears to improve and the child begins to gain weight excessively to well above the 50th percentile for weight.[26] In our study several mothers reported that this weight increase occurred before the second stage in which appetite becomes excessive and food foraging behaviour begins. At present this change in weight and its relationship to feeding is poorly understood.

There is some variation in the age at which parents first become aware of the excessive interest in food, and also in the associated food seeking behaviour. With some children, families report that from the time the child becomes more mobile and can seek out food it is necessary to lock food away at all times. Other families report that some children or adults with PWS appeared to control their own food input successfully while living at home or in supervised settings. However, parents were always watchful and none thought their son or daughter could live a totally independent life with full control of their own food intake. In support of parental observations are the studies of eating behaviour in experimental settings that have found that eating continues for the majority of those with PWS whilst food remains available.[27,28] Stomach surgery, such as gastric bypass operations,[29] has been used in the past to try to reduce gross obesity, but without also having control of access to food it has only been temporarily successful. A trial of fenfluramine, an appetite suppressive medication, has also proved ineffective in reducing food intake.[30]

In research going back over 20 years, it has been shown that the food requirements of people with PWS are less than those of all comparison groups tested, possibly due in part to their apparent aversion to exercise, as well as their abnormal body composition. This low calorie requirement naturally exacerbates the tendency to obesity caused by the insatiable appetite. However, the only reliable way to maintain a healthy weight in people with PWS is to significantly restrict food intake, for example, by controlling access to food. This has raised ethical questions with regard to adults with PWS,[31,32] and it may be argued that a fundamental right is violated by controlling access to food. However, there is a convincing argument that people with PWS lack the capacity to make decisions about eating for themselves even though they may have the capacity to make many other decisions in their lives.[31,33,34]

The obesity originally described by Prader *et al.* as being a central feature of the syndrome therefore appears to have two components. First, there is a marked propensity to over-eat and a failure to limit calorie intake and, second, a low level of calorie expenditure. The basis for the eating behaviour has been investigated behaviourally and with respect to possible central and/or peripherally pathophysiological mechanisms.

The question arises as to whether the drive to eat is a fault of the hunger drive over-riding a normal satiety response, that is, the person feels full yet continues to eat, or that the satiation response is impaired, so that the person never feels full. There is quite convincing evidence that the latter is the case.[27] Behavioural, cognitive and metabolic responses to food intake were studied in 13 adults with PWS and 10 age-matched controls. Using sandwich quarters, standardised to provide 51.6 kcal with 4.1 g protein, 7.8 g carbohydrates, 1.78 g fat and 1.56 g fibre, rates of eating were observed during one hour's access to food and feelings of hunger were assessed using a visual analogue scale. Blood was taken for estimation of glucose, insulin, cholecystokinin (CCK), prolactin, growth hormone and cortisol every 20 minutes for a total period of 100 minutes. Ten of the PWS group ate steadily for the whole hour that food was available and on average consumed three times more calories than the comparison group. The median ratings for feelings of hunger in the PWS group changed in the expected direction but were delayed compared with those of the comparison group, and only reached the same levels as those in the comparison group after those with PWS had eaten a significantly greater amount of food. In contrast to the comparison group, feelings of hunger in the PWS group were reported to re-emerge shortly after food was removed. Increases in plasma glucose levels were inversely correlated with changes in hunger ratings in the PWS group, but not in the comparison group. There was a significantly greater increase in serum CCK levels during the meal in the PWS group than in the comparison group, indicating that, in PWS, failure of peripheral release of CCK in response to food intake was not the explanation for the impaired satiety response. Other studies have also shown increased food intake by people with PWS in experimental conditions with only relatively modest influence of naloxone or pancreatic polypeptide infusions[35, 36] on this behaviour. These earlier studies did not investigate hunger and satiety. From a behavioural perspective, it therefore seems likely that there is an impaired and insensitive satiety response to food intake and that continuing feelings of hunger, which only briefly diminish following significant calorie intake, drive the over-eating behaviour. What then is the basis for this apparent abnormality of the satiety response to food intake?

Neuroendocrine and gut hormone studies in PWS

Most adults maintain an amazingly stable energy balance between the body's energy expenditure and the intake of food over long time periods so as to maintain a fairly constant body weight. This is despite the wide fluctuations in daily food intake and energy expenditure. The exact mechanisms that underlie this energy balance are

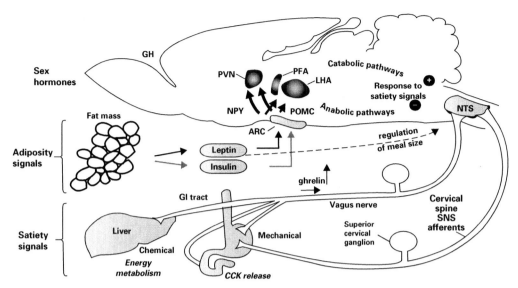

Figure 2.1.   Hunger and satiety signalling between body and brain. NPY, neuropeptide Y; POMC, proopiomelanocortin; CCK, cholecystokinin; GH, growth hormone; PVN, paraventricular nucleus; PFA, perifornical area; LHA, lateral hypothalamic area; NTS, nucleus of the solitary tract; ARC, arcuate nucleus; GI tract, gastro-intestinal tract; SNS, sensory nervous system.

not yet understood, but animal experiments have implicated certain brain areas, notably the hypothalamus and hindbrain, and certain neurotransmitters and their receptors as having important roles in the process.

One such animal model is the creation of the obese ob/ob mouse.[37] This breed of mouse has a genetically determined lack of the hormone leptin. Furthermore, a small number of people have been described with early onset severe obesity as a result of over-eating that have been shown to have a genetically-determined lack of leptin[38] or a leptin receptor abnormality.[39] In the case of the former, leptin replacement results in reduction in eating and loss of weight.[40] These observations prompted several investigations of leptin levels in people with PWS. [25,41,42,43] In PWS, plasma levels of leptin have been shown to correlate with percentage body fat as found in the general population.[43] Moreover, after a year of treatment with growth hormone, both plasma leptin and percentage body fat were reduced, again as would be predicted. Whilst these studies cannot rule out the possibility of a leptin receptor deficit in PWS, they do indicate that leptin deficiency cannot account for the eating behaviour.

A fairly simple outline model of the mechanisms that control energy balance, consistent with animal studies and studies of normal people, has been proposed.[44] This is shown schematically in Figure 2.1. Signals from fat stores in the body are carried by insulin and leptin (and maybe other hormones), to the hypothalamus where they act on central effector pathways. When fat levels are high, these signals repress brain anabolic neural circuits that stimulate eating and inhibit energy expenditure, while simultaneously stimulating catabolic circuits that inhibit food intake and increase energy expenditure. When fat levels are low, the signals carried by insulin and leptin stimulate anabolic neural pathways and suppress catabolic pathways. Leptin/insulin-sensitive central effector pathways also interact with hindbrain satiety circuits to regulate onset of satiety and thus control meal size, rather than meal frequency, to achieve energy balance. Since fat stores change relatively slowly, these tend to be long-term effects, and leptin appears to be the more important regulatory hormone.

On a daily basis, eating onset is governed by short-term factors (e.g. time of day, emotional state, availability and palatability of food, etc.). The ingestion of food generates neural and hormonal satiety signals to the hindbrain and eating ceases. In particular, it seems that one way in which hunger is signalled is by the secretion of the hormone ghrelin from the stomach to the hindbrain. After the ingestion of food, ghrelin levels fall.[44,45,46] In PWS, in line with the excess fat mass, leptin levels are high[47] and anabolic neural circuits appear to be repressed, in that neuropeptide Y (NPY) levels are low and agouti-related protein (AGRP) levels unchanged.[48] We would therefore expect that meal size would decrease to balance the long-term energy needs. However, unlike other obese groups, ghrelin levels remain high and may therefore continue to stimulate eating.[46] This failure of calorie intake to lead to a fall in ghrelin levels could be an important mechanism causing the eating disturbance in PWS. However, the cause of the apparent over-production of ghrelin in PWS is not known (but see Chapter 12) and it may only be an epiphenomenon reflecting the presence of a fundamental deficit elsewhere in the feedback loop.

The hormone ghrelin not only plays a role in eating behaviour, it also stimulates the release of growth hormone. We should therefore expect high levels of growth hormone in PWS. Normally, as indicated above, ghrelin is produced in response to hunger and levels fall again when hunger is satisfied, so that stimulation of growth hormone release occurs in discrete episodes. However, in rats, continuous stimulation by ghrelin causes growth hormone release to fall back over time as a result of receptor desensitisation.[49] If this also occurs in humans, it could reconcile the observed low levels of growth hormone with continuously high levels of ghrelin.

Sleep

Sleep disturbance, night-time disturbance, or sleep abnormality and/or daytime sleepiness, is one of the clinical diagnostic features of PWS. The connection between sleep disturbance and daytime sleepiness has been investigated in a number of studies. In the Cambridge study, according to parent/carer reports, it was concluded that a sleep disturbance probably contributed to daytime sleepiness in some, but by no means all, people with the syndrome (see Chapter 9). A questionnaire study of 29 people with PWS and an age and gender matched comparison group reported similar sleep disturbances to those of the Cambridge study. There were more sleep problems in the PWS group compared with the comparison group, and no association between sleep problems and body mass index or weight.[50]

More sophisticated measures, such as polysomnographic recordings and multiple sleep latency tests have been used over the last decade in studies of sleep in PWS. In some of these studies it is not clear how PWS was diagnosed and numbers of people studied have varied, but, in general, findings have been consistent[51,52,53,54,55,56,57]. As long ago as 1993, a study of 15 adults and nine children with PWS[57] found little or no sleep apnoea in their sample, but frequent rapid eye movement (REM) related oxygen desaturation, the severity of which correlated with increased obesity. Abnormal REM sleep cycles with variable REM latency, and fragmented REM sleep with multiple brief REM periods were observed in both adults and children. Rapid eye movement sleep abnormalities were found in some people without REM related oxygen desaturisation. In the same year, in a study of 21 people with PWS and 19 people without PWS,[56] excessive daytime sleepiness was found in 95% of the PWS group and REM sleep disorders (sleep onset REMs, REM sleep in naps, many arousals during REM sleep, significant decrease in total REM sleep) in 52%. No sleep apnoea was found in this sample of people with PWS, unlike other studies.[51,52,53] A study of arousal and cardio-respiratory responses to hypoxia in people with PWS found both to be abnormal, with only one of 13 in the PWS group, but seven of 11 in the comparison group being aroused by the hypoxic challenge.[55] Heart rate increased significantly less in the PWS group. Respiratory rate did not change, but did increase by 13% in those in the comparison group. In one study, five of seven obese people with PWS who were considered to have symptomatic sleep apnoea were treated with continuous positive airway pressure over a six-month period. Excessive daytime sleepiness persisted in two and improved in three of these people.[52]

Temperature

Two types of temperature abnormalities have been reported in PWS. First, actual body temperature and, second, perception of temperature. PWS babies often have difficulty with body temperature regulation, but most adapt as they get older. A few older people with PWS have more severe difficulties, such as a man, reported at the Third Triennial International PWS Conference, who became comatose when body temperature dropped to 81 °F (*c.* 27 °C). Several other such examples were reported at that same conference. Poor temperature perception is more common. In the Cambridge study, several adults were not allowed to run their own bathwater because they could not judge the temperature safely (see also Chapter 9). Quite a few have some mild symptoms, such as wearing clothing unsuited to the season of year (heavy wool jumpers in summer or thin T-shirts in winter). Body temperature in children with PWS was investigated in a postal questionnaire study[58] that asked about the frequency of occurrence of temperatures above 104 °F (c. 38 °C) and 105 °F (c. 38.5 °C), related to and unrelated to illness, and of temperatures below 94 °F (c. 34.5 °C). Comparison groups comprised siblings of the PWS group, children with other neurodevelopmental problems and normal healthy children matched to the PWS group for age and gender. Significant differences were found between the PWS group and both sibling and normal comparison groups in the prevalence of febrile convulsions (5.9% v. 0%), fever associated symptoms (12.9% v. 3.5%) and temperatures below 94 °F / c. 34.5 °C (8.2% v. 0%). There were no differences between the PWS and neurodevelopmentally impaired groups, which was interpreted as evidence against a specific PWS involvement. Faulty regulation of temperature by the hypothalamus is thought to be responsible for these phenomena.

High pain threshold

A higher proportion of people with learning disabilities, compared to the normal population, seem to have raised pain thresholds. This is observed to an even greater extent in people with PWS. In the Cambridge study some extreme examples were reported (see also Chapter 9). For example, there was a young man who went to work with a broken ankle. A young boy, who having been seriously injured by a swing while playing, carried on until teatime, his mother discovering his broken arm hanging limply when she removed his coat. Similarly, another boy with a perforated bowel only complained of a slight ache. Such examples, and similar ones from other researchers, have led to calls for vigilance and investigation of even mild complaints of feeling unwell when made by people with PWS. Self-harm, usually in the form of skin picking, is also common in PWS, and it is thought that the maintenance of this behaviour may be partly contributed to by the presence of a high pain threshold. This is especially true where there is a pre-existing scar such as that of the man whose operation scar, sustained seven years previously, had still not healed because of his constant picking.

It is not clear whether people with PWS actually feel less pain or whether their interpretation of the sensation of painful stimuli is different – that is, whether the differences between their responses and those of the general population are physiological or cognitive. One study looked at somatosensory functions in five children aged 11–13 years with PWS.[59] It was found that tactual perception in the hands was apparently normal in four of them and that sensory nerve conduction velocities in the median nerve and latencies for sensory evoked potentials in PWS were similar to those of 10 children without PWS. Thus there appeared to be a preserved myelinisation of sensory nerve fibres in PWS. However, sensory nerve action potentials in the PWS group averaged, at most, half of normal size, suggesting a reduced number of normal axons in the median nerve. Similar neurographic findings and a low density of peripheral nerve fibres have been reported in people with hereditary or congenital insensitivity to pain.[60] Regulation of pain is mediated through the hypothalamus and a deficit in the hypothalamus is one possible explanation of the raised pain threshold.

Imaging and pathological studies of the brain in PWS

One of the early reports using magnetic resonance imaging (MRI) to look at brain morphology and involving a person with PWS was the investigation of patients with disorders of the hypothalamo-pituitary area.[61] The person with PWS was included as one of six people with hypogonadotrophic hypogonadism. The sellar area was reported as normal in all six participants (one with PWS). In an MRI study of four people with PWS and six with Angelman syndrome (AS), the length of the banks of the Sylvian fissure in a gapless series of thin sagittal images was investigated.[62] The authors reported that 12% of those with PWS had anomalous fissures, as opposed to 75% in those with AS. They speculated that this observation might account for the severe language disorder found in people with AS. A study motivated by the growth hormone deficiency in PWS used MRI to investigate the site of growth hormone synthesis in the anterior pituitary gland.[63] The authors found no statistically significant difference in the height of the anterior pituitary gland in the 15 children with PWS studied, compared with children either from the general population or those with isolated growth hormone deficiency. However, they noted the curious finding that the posterior pituitary bright spot was absent in three of the PWS group and decreased in size in a fourth.

More recently, in a proton magnetic resonance spectroscopy study of the brains of five people with PWS and 37 in a comparison group, it was reported that the MRI revealed mild abnormalities in all cases.[64] These abnormalities consisted of: ventriculomegaly (four people); mild frontal cortical atrophy (three people); delayed myelination (one person); and a small brainstem (one person). The study also looked at relationships between several metabolites that can be detected in the human brain and IQ or developmental levels. The metabolites were: N-acetylaspartate (NAA); choline (Cho); creatine (Cr); and lactate. No peaks were observed for lactate and, in the PWS group, the peak for NAA tended to be small. In keeping with this, the ratios NAA/Cho and NAA/Cr were smaller in PWS than in the comparison group, but Cho/Cr did not differ. In the PWS group the correlations of IQ with both NAA/Cho and Cho/Cr were significant. The authors concluded that NAA may be decreased in the brains of people with PWS and that, since NAA is present in neurones and appears to be a valid indicator of neurone functioning, there may be neurone loss or neurone dysfunction in PWS.

Another non-invasive technique for studying brain activity – event-related potentials (in response to unexpected stimuli) extracted from the electroencephalogram – was used in a study of 10 people with PWS and 10 control adults.[65] The unexpected stimulus typically elicits a positive event-related potential (P3) with maximum amplitude at centro-parietal scalp sites and with a latency of roughly 300 ms from stimulus onset. Similar visual and auditory tasks were used to detect modality effects. In both tasks, P3 was deflated relative to those in a comparison group, but more so in the auditory modality. The authors concluded that short-term memory is impaired in PWS and that the visual modality is less affected than the auditory modality.

The need for pathological studies of the brains of people with PWS was mentioned at the beginning of this chapter, and the final studies to be described report on what has already been done. The earliest is the study of the hypothalamic paraventricular nucleus in the brains of five people who had PWS and the brains of 27 from a comparison group donated to the centre cited in connection with this work.[66] The paraventricular nucleus (PVN) was morphometrically investigated after conventional staining with thionine and immunocytochemical staining for oxytocin (OXT) and arginine vasopressin (AVP). The thionine-stained volume of the PVN was 28% smaller in the PWS group and the total cell number was 38% lower. The immunoreactivity for OXT and AVP was decreased in the PWS group but variability within both groups was high. A significant decrease of 42% in the number of OXT-expressing neurones was found in the PWS group and the volume of the PVN containing such neurones was decreased by 54%. The number of AVP-expressing neurones in the PVN was not significantly different for the two groups. The authors concluded that the OXT neurones of the PVN seem to be good candidates for playing a physiological role in eating behaviour as "satiety neurones" in the human hypothalamus. On the other hand, elevated levels of OXT but similar levels of AVP have been reported in the cerebrospinal fluid in five people with PWS compared with six in a comparison group.[67] These two studies show the importance of measurements made in the brain, rather than in other body locations when trying to elucidate brain–behaviour links. Two further published studies of the brains of deceased people with PWS are important. The first followed-up a previous finding concerning the neuroendocrine chaperone 7B2, whose gene is located in 15q13–14

Table 2.1. Key findings from investigations of biological and regulatory mechanisms in Prader–Willi syndrome (PWS)

1. Abnormalities of eating, growth, sexual development, as well as temperature regulation, sleep and insensitivity to pain, characteristic of people with PWS support the view that in PWS there is an abnormality of hypothalamic function.
2. Reduction in hypothalamic oxytocin containing neurones in PWS has been suggested as a potential explanation for the abnormal eating behaviour, but whether or not this is the fundamental deficit that accounts for the eating behaviour is, as yet, unknown. Other abnormalities, such as the initiation of labour by a baby with PWS, suggest that oxytocin deficit may be important.
3. Levels of leptin are as expected in relationship to fat mass. Other than abnormalities of oxytocin containing neurones, no central neurotransmitter abnormality has been found that might account for the eating behaviour. Persistent high levels in the blood of the gut orexigenic hormone ghrelin in people with PWS might account for the eating behaviour.

adjacent to the PWS region on chromosome 15.[68] 7B2 immunoreactivity in the supraoptic nucleus (SON) or the PVN had been found in only three of the five PWS brains investigated. In the follow-up, the same two PWS brains also failed to show any reaction using two antibodies directed against processed vasopressin (VP). However, all PWS brains reacted normally with five antibodies that recognise different parts of the VP precursor. The authors concluded that there was therefore a processing deficit in the two abnormal cases. Further investigation, determining the expression of the neuroendocrine convertases PC1 and PC2 in the SON and PVN hypothalamic cells, showed that the two anomalous PWS cases had no PC2 immunoreactivity, but PC1 immunoreactivity was only slightly diminished. Thus, in the VP neurones of two PWS brains, greatly reduced amounts of 7B2 and PC2 were present, resulting in diminished VP precursor processing. In a second study[48] in an attempt to identify causes of leptin resistance in human obesity, NPY and AGRP neurones were examined in the hypothalami of the post-mortem brains of people with and without PWS, and other obese people. NPY and AGRP were co-localised in infundibular neurones. NPY immunocytochemistry staining and mRNA expression were reduced in the brains of the obese groups but AGRP immunocytochemistry staining was unchanged, suggesting normal responses of NPY and AGRP neurones to peripheral signals, such as leptin and insulin in human obesity, including PWS.

In Table 2.1 we have listed some of the key findings that have come from biological research and from the investigation of the hypothalamic based regulatory systems of the body. Much of what is observed can be putatively traced back to hypothalamic dysfunction. Ultimately the cognitive and behavioural findings need to be mapped to these and other pathophysiological mechanisms. This is discussed in later chapters of the book.

REFERENCES

1. Leibowitz, S. F., Hammer, N. J. & Chang, K. Hypothalamic paraventricular nucleus lesions produce overeating and obesity in the rat. *Physiology and Behaviour* **27** (1981), 1031–1040.
2. Rogers, R. C. & Hermann, G. E. Oxytocin, oxytocin antagonist, TRH, and hypothalamic paraventricular nucleus stimulation effects on gastric motility. *Peptides* **8** (1986), 505–513.
3. Williams, G., Bing, C., Cai, X. J. *et al.* The hypothalamus and the control of energy homeostasis: different circuits, different purposes. *Physiology & Behaviour* **74** (2001), 683–701.
4. Buijs, R. M., De Vries, G. J., Van Leeuwen, F. W. & Swaab, D. F. Vasopressin and oxytocin: distribution and putative functions in the brain. In Cross, B. A. & Leng, G. A. (Eds). The neurohypophysis: structure, function and control. *Progress in Brain Research* **60** (1983), 115–122.
5. Blundell, J. E., Lawton, C. L. & Hill, A. J. Mechanisms of appetite control and their abnormalities in obese patients. *Hormone Research* **39** Suppl. 3 (1993), 72–76.
6. Swaab D. F. Prader–Willi syndrome and the hypothalamus. *Acta Paediatrica Supplement* **423** (1997), 50–54.
7. Wharton, R. H. & Bresman, M. J. Neonatal respiratory depression and delay in diagnosis in Prader–Willi syndrome. *Developmental Medicine and Child Neurology* **31** (1989), 231–236.
8. Swaab, D. F., Boer, K. & Honnebier, W. J. The influence of the fetal hypothalamus and pituitary on the onset and course of parturition. In Knight, J. & O'Connor, M. (Eds). *The Fetus and Birth. Ciba Foundation Symposium* 47, pp. 379–400. Amsterdam, New York: Elsevier/North Holland Biomedical Press 1977.
9. Willnow, S., Kiess, W., Butenandt, O. *et al.* Endocrine disorders in septo-optic dysplasia (De Morsier syndrome) – evaluation and follow up of 18 patients. *European Journal of Pediatrics* **155** (1996), 179–184.
10. Schulze, A., Mogensen, H., Hamborg-Petersen, B. *et al.* Fertility in Prader–Willi syndrome: a case report with Angelman syndrome in the offspring. *Acta Paediatrica* **90** (2001), 455–459.
11. Akefeldt, A., Tornhage, C. J. & Gillberg, C. 'A woman with Prader–Willi syndrome gives birth to a healthy baby girl'. *Developmental Medicine and Child Neurology* **41** (1999), 789–790.
12. Jeffcoate, W. J., Laurance, B. M., Edwards, C. R. & Besser, G. M. Endocrine function in the Prader–Willi syndrome. *Clinical Endocrinology* (Oxf), **12** (1980), 81–89.
13. Gillessen-Kaesbach, G., Robinson, W., Lohmann, D., Kaya-Westerloh, S., Passarge, E. & Horsthemke, B. Genotype-phenotype correlation in a series of 167 deletion and non-deletion patients with Prader–Willi syndrome. *Human Genetics* **96** (1995), 638–643.
14. Butler, M. G. & Meaney, F. J. Standards for selected anthropometric measurements in Prader–Willi syndrome. *Pediatrics*, **88** (1991), 853–860.
15. Grugni, G., Guzzaloni, G., Moro, D., Bettio, D., De Medici, C. & Morabito, F. Reduced growth hormone (GH) responsiveness to combined GH-releasing hormone and pyridostigmine administration in the Prader–Willi syndrome. *Clinical Endocrinology* **48** (1998), 769–775.

16. Carrel, A. L., Myers, S. E., Whitman, B. Y. & Allen, D. B. Growth hormone improves body composition, fat utilization, physical strength and agility, and growth in Prader–Willi syndrome: a controlled study. *Journal of Pediatrics* **134** (1999), 215–221.

17. Davies, P. S. W., Evans, S., Broomhead, S. *et al.* Effect of growth hormone on height, weight, and body composition in Prader–Willi syndrome. *Archives of Disease in Childhood* **78** (1998), 474–476.

18. Lindgren, A. C., Hagenas, L., Muller, J. *et al.* Growth hormone treatment of children with Prader–Willi syndrome affects linear growth and body composition favourably. *Acta Paediatrica* **87** (1998), 28–31.

19. Whitman, B. Y. & Myers, S. *A two year treatment/control group study of growth hormone replacement therapy: results at one year.* Paper presented at the 4th triennial IPWSO scientific conference 2001, Saint Paul, Minnesota, USA.

20. Van Mil, E. G., Westerterp, K. R., Kester, A. D. *et al.* Activity related energy expenditure in children and adolescents with Prader–Willi syndrome. *International Journal of Obesity and Related Metabolic Disorders* **24** (2000), 429–434.

21. Davis, P. S. W. & Joughlin, C. Using stable isotopes to assess reduced physical activity of individuals with Prader–Willi syndrome. *American Journal of Mental Retardation* **98** (1993), 349–353.

22. Brynes, A., Goldstone, A. P., Thomas, E. L. *et al. Unusual body composition in Prader–Willi syndrome explains reduced resting metabolic rate.* Paper presented at the 3rd triennial IPWSO scientific conference 1998, Venice, Italy.

23. Schoeller, D. A., Levitsky, L. L., Bandini, L. G., Dietz, W. W. & Walczak, A. Energy expenditure and body composition in Prader–Willi syndrome. *Metabolism* **37** (1988), 115–120.

24. Brambilla, P., Bosio, L., Manzoni, P., Pietrobelli, A., Beccaria, L. & Chiumello, G. Peculiar body composition in patients with Prader–Labhart–Willi syndrome. *American Journal of Clinical Nutrition* **65** (1997), 1369–1374.

25. Eiholzer, U., Blum, W. F. & Molinari, L. Body fat determined by skinfold measurements is elevated despite underweight in infants with Prader–Labhart–Willi syndrome. *Journal of Pediatrics* **134** (1999), 222–225.

26. Greenswag, L. R. Adults with Prader–Willi syndrome: a survey of 232 cases. *Developmental Medicine and Child Neurology* **29** (1987), 145–152.

27. Holland, A. J., Treasure, J., Coskeran, P., Dallow, J., Milton, N. & Hillhouse, E. Measurement of excessive appetite and metabolic changes in Prader–Willi syndrome. *International Journal of Obesity* **17** (1993), 526–532.

28. Lindgren, A. C., Barkeling, B., Hagg, A., Ritzen, E. M., Marcus, C. & Rossner, S. Eating behavior in Prader–Willi syndrome, normal weight, and obese control groups. *Journal of Pediatrics* **137** (2000), 50–55.

29. Soper, R. T., Mason, E. E., Printen, K. J. & Zellweger, H. Surgical treatment of morbid obesity in Prader–Willi syndrome. In Holm, V. A., Sulzbacher, S. J. & Pipes, P. L. (Eds). *The Prader–Willi syndrome.* Baltimore: University Park Press, 1981.

30. Selikowitz, M., Sunman, J., Pendergast, A. & Wright, S. Fenfluramine in Prader–Willi syndrome: a double blind, placebo controlled trial. *Archives of Disease in Childhood* **65** (1990), 112–114.

31. Holland, A. J. & Wong, J. Genetically determined obesity in Prader–Willi syndrome: the ethics and legality of treatment. *Journal of Medical Ethics* **25** (1999), 230–236.

32. Dykens, E. M., Goff, B. J., Hodapp, R. M. *et al.* Eating themselves to death: have 'personal rights' gone too far in treating people with Prader–Willi syndrome? *Mental Retardation* **35** (1997), 312–314.

33. Holland, A. J. Understanding the eating disorder affecting people with Prader–Willi syndrome. *Journal of Applied Research in Intellectual Disorders* **11** (1998), 192–206.

34. Van Hooren, R. H., Widdershoven, G. A. M., van den Borne, H. W. & Curfs, L. M. G. Autonomy and intellectual disability: the case of prevention of obesity in Prader–Willi syndrome. *Journal of Intellectual Disability Research* **46** (2002), 560–568.

35. Hayward, M. D. & Low M. J. The effect of naloxone on operant behavior for food reinforcers in DBA/2 mice. *Brain Research Bulletin* **56** (2001), 537–543.

36. Batterham, R. L., Le Roux, C. W., Cohen, M. A. *et al.* Pancreatic polypeptide reduces appetite and food intake in humans. *Journal of Clinical Endocrinology and Metabolism* **88** (2003), 3989–3992.

37. Bray, G. A. Hereditary adiposity in mice: human lessons from the yellow and obese (OB/OB) mice. *Obesity Research* **4** (1996), 91–95.

38. Montague, C. T., Farooqi, I. S., Whitehead, J. P. *et al.* Congenital leptin deficiency is associated with severe early-onset obesity in humans. *Nature* **387** (1997), 903–908.

39. Clement, K., Vaisse, C., Lahlou, N. *et al.* A mutation in the human leptin receptor gene causes obesity and pituitary dysfunction. *Nature* **392** (1998), 398–401.

40. Farooqi, I. S., Matarese, G., Lord, G. M. *et al.* Beneficial effects of leptin on obesity, T cell hyporesponsiveness, and neuroendocrine/metabolic dysfunction of human congenital leptin deficiency. *Journal of Clinical Investigation* **110** (2002), 1093–1103.

41. Elimam, A., Lindgren, A. C., Norgren, S. *et al.* Growth hormone treatment downregulates serum leptin levels in children independent of changes in body mass index. *Hormone Research* **52** (1999), 66–72.

42. Myers, S. E., Davis, A., Whitman, B. Y., Santiago, J. V. and Landt, M. Leptin concentrations in Prader–Willi syndrome before and after growth hormone replacement. *Clinical Endocrinology* **52** (2000), 101–105.

43. Goldstone, A. P., Brynes, A. E., Thomas, E. L. *et al.* Resting metabolic rate, plasma leptin concentrations, leptin receptor expression, and adipose tissue measured by whole-body magnetic resonance imaging in women with Prader–Willi syndrome. *American Journal of Clinical Nutrition* **75** (2002), 468–475.

44. Schwartz M. W., Woods, S. C., Porte, D. Jr, Seeley, R. J. & Baskin, D. G. Central nervous system control of food intake. *Nature* **404** (2000), 661–670.

45. Kojima, M., Hosoda, H., Date, Y., Nakazato, M., Matsuo, H. & Kangawa, K. Ghrelin is a growth-hormone-releasing acylated peptide from stomach. *Nature* **402** (1999), 656–660.

46. DelParigi, A., Tschop, M., Heiman, M. L. *et al.* High circulating ghrelin: a potential cause for hyperphagia and obesity in Prader–Willi syndrome. *Journal of Clinical Endocrinology and Metabolism* **87** (2002), 5461–5464.

47. Goldstone, A. P., Brynes, A. E. & Thoma, E. L. Resting metabolic rate, plasma leptin concentrations, leptin receptor expression, and adipose tissue measured by whole-body magnetic

resonance imaging in women with Prader–Willi syndrome. *American Journal of Clinical Nutrition* **75** (2002), 468–475.

48. Goldstone, A. P., Unmehopa, U. A., Bloom, S. R. & Swaab, D. F. Hypothalamic NPY and agouti-related protein are increased in human illness but not in Prader–Willi syndrome and other obese subjects. *Journal of Clinical Endocrinology and Metabolism* **87** (2002), 927–937.

49. Date, Y., Murakami, N., Kojima, M. *et al.* Central effects of a novel acylated peptide, ghrelin, on growth hormone release in rats. *Biochemical and Biophysical Research Communications* **275** (2000), 477–480.

50. Richdale, A. L., Cotton, S. & Hibbit, K. Sleep and behaviour disturbance in Prader–Willi syndrome: a questionnaire study. *Journal of Intellectual Disability Research* **43** (1999), 380–392.

51. Manni, R., Politini, L., Nobili, L. *et al.* Hypersomnia in the Prader–Willi syndrome: clinical-electrophysiological features and underlying factors. *Clinical Neurophysiology* **112** (2001), 800–805.

52. Clift, S., Dahlitz, M. & Parkes, J. D. Sleep apnoea in the Prader–Willi syndrome. *Journal of Sleep Research* **3** (1994), 121–126.

53. Schluter, B., Buschatz, D., Trowitzsch, E., Aksu, F. & Andler, W. Respiratory control in children with Prader–Willi syndrome. *European Journal of Pediatrics* **156** (1997), 65–68.

54. Vgontzas, A. N., Bixler, E. O., Kales, A. *et al.* Daytime sleepiness and REM abnormalities in Prader–Willi syndrome: evidence of generalized hypoarousal. *International Journal of Neuroscience* **87** (1996), 127–139.

55. Arens, R., Gozal, D., Burrell, B. C. *et al.* Arousal and cardiorespiratory responses to hypoxia in Prader–Willi syndrome. *American Journal of Respiratory Critical Care Medicine* **153** (1996), 283–287.

56. Helbing-Zwanenburg, B., Kamphuisen, H. A. & Mourtazaev, M. S. The origin of excessive daytime sleepiness in the Prader–Willi syndrome. *Journal of Intellectual Disability Research* **37** (1993), 533–541.

57. Hertz, G., Cataletto, M., Feinsilver, S. H. & Angulo, M. Sleep and breathing patterns in patients with Prader–Willi syndrome (PWS): effects of age and gender. *Sleep* **16** (1993), 366–371.

58. Williams, M. S., Rooney, B. L., Williams, J., Josephson, K. & Pauli, R. Investigation of thermoregulatory characteristics in patients With Prader–Willi syndrome. *American Journal of Medical Genetics* **49** (1994), 302–307.

59. Brandt, B. R. & Rosen, I. Impaired peripheral somatosensory function in children with Prader–Willi syndrome. *Neuropediatrics* **29** (1998), 124–126.

60. Karkashan, E. M., Joharji, H. S. & Al-Harbi, N. N. Congenital insensitivity to pain in four related Saudi families. *Pediatric Dermatology* **19** (2002), 333–335.

61. Cacciari, E., Zucchini, S., Carla, G. *et al.* Endocrine function and morphological findings in patients with disorders of the hypothalamo-pituitary area: a study with magnetic resonance. *Archives of Disease in Childhood* **65** (1990), 1199–1202.

62. Leonard, C. M., Williams, C. A., Nicholls, R. D. *et al.* Angelman and Prader–Willi syndromes: a magnetic resonance imaging study of differences in cerebral structure. *American Journal of Medical Genetics* **46** (1993), 26–33.

63. Miller, L., Angulo, M., Price, D. & Taneja, S. MR of the pituitary in patients with Prader–Willi syndrome: size determination and imaging findings. *Pediatric Radiology* **26** (1996), 43–47.

64. Hashimoto, T., Mori, K., Yoneda, Y. *et al.* Proton magnetic resonance spectroscopy of the brain in patients with Prader–Willi syndrome. *Pediatric Neurology* **18** (1998), 30–35.

65. Stauder, J. E., Brinkman, M. J. & Curfs, L. M. Multi-modal P3 deflation of event-related brain activity in Prader–Willi syndrome. *Neuroscience Letters* **327** (2002), 99–102.

66. Swaab, D. F., Purba, J. S. & Hofman, M. A. Alterations in the hypothalamic paraventricular nucleus and its oxytocin neurones (putative satiety cells) in Prader–Willi syndrome: a study of five cases. *Journal of Clinical Endocrinology and Metabolism* **80** (1995), 573–579.

67. Martin, A., State, M., Anderson, G. M. *et al.* Cerebrospinal fluid levels of oxytocin in Prader–Willi syndrome: a preliminary report. *Biological Psychiatry* **44** (1998), 1349–1352.

68. Gabreels, B. A., Swaab, D. F., de Kleijn, D. P. *et al.* Attenuation of the polypeptide 7B2, prohormone convertase PC2, and vasopressin in the hypothalamus of some Prader–Willi patients: indications for a processing defect. *Journal of Clinical Endocrinology and Metabolism* **83** (1998), 591–599.

3

The Cambridge PWS project

The need for a population survey

At the Third Triennial International PWS Conference in Venice in 1998, the scientists present agreed that a large population prevalence study of PWS was needed for two main reasons. First, the two earlier population surveys had not been large enough to produce reliable estimates and, in the case of one of them that surveyed people aged 0–25 years, had not been comprehensive. Moreover, neither of these two studies used genetic criteria for the diagnosis of PWS and therefore the prevalences were very likely to be over-estimates. A larger population study, using established clinical diagnostic criteria together with recently agreed genetic diagnostic techniques, would therefore provide more accurate population prevalence and birth incidence figures. Second, the possibility of sampling bias could not be ruled out where conflicting findings had been obtained in different studies that used groups of people with PWS who were ascertained via specialist clinics or who had volunteered. It was strongly suspected that such a bias was an explanation for at least some of the contradictions. That is, in these conflicting studies, the groups of people with PWS who were included were probably not representative of the PWS population more generally. A new population survey, with genetic confirmation of the diagnosis, would both provide a representative sample of people with PWS to help with future research and more accurate prevalence data on which to determine service requirements.

Aims of the project

The two main aims of the Cambridge project were to identify all people with PWS living in what was then the Anglia & Oxford Health Region, and to investigate the full range of the PWS phenotype in that population-based group of people who were ascertained to have PWS. The Anglia & Oxford Health Region consisted of the counties of Bedfordshire, Berkshire, Buckinghamshire, Cambridgeshire, Norfolk,

Northamptonshire, Oxfordshire and Suffolk, with a combined total population of a little over five million (5 044 233 at the 1991 census). The size of the region studied was chosen after administrative and statistical considerations. Using a health region is advantageous administratively, since ethics committees and laboratory and clinical facilities are region-based. Previously published prevalence figures suggested that there might be as many as 200–300 people with PWS in the Region.

Finding people with PWS

Given the size of the population and the probable low prevalence rate of PWS, a complete screening of everyone in that population for possible PWS was not practicable or appropriate. The only practical ascertainment methodology was to search for people with possible PWS by various means and assume that all the population not seen did not have PWS. For the purposes of the initial identification and in order to ensure as far as possible that no people with PWS were missed, an over-inclusive criterion was adopted. Everyone was included who was reported to possibly have PWS or who had five or more of the following nine symptoms: extreme floppiness at birth; initial failure to thrive or difficulty in feeding after birth; the development of severe over-eating and/or rapid weight gain in early childhood; obesity or the need for weight control; problems with sexual development (e.g. undescended testes, delayed periods); some learning disability (mental handicap); small hands and feet; short stature or the need for growth hormone; and an abnormality of chromosome 15.

The search was conducted through groups and professionals who might come into contact with people with PWS and initially included: the PWSA (UK); all those in relevant genetics departments; paediatricians who were registered members of the Royal College of Paediatricians; paediatricians who were listed in the Anglia & Oxford Health Region Handbook; psychiatrists in learning disabilities who were registered members of the Royal College of Psychiatrists; and psychiatrists in learning disabilities who were listed in the Anglia & Oxford Health Region Handbook. There was some debate as to whether or not General Practitioners (GPs) should be included in this list. Eventually it was decided to write to all known GPs in the Cambridge area only, in order to see how cost effective this strategy might be. No new cases were identified, although several were confirmed, and this strategy was abandoned. The next groups of professionals contacted were: dieticians; community nurses; and those working in Local authority departments dealing with Special Education and Social Services and, through them, special schools for people with learning disabilities and residential homes for people with learning disabilities. Finally, an attempt was made to contact parents and carers through appeals in the media, including newspapers, television and radio, using the same screening criteria as above. For the purposes of prevalence estimation, it was decided, prior to the start of the population study, not to include all those people with PWS living in a specialist group of homes for people with PWS located in the Health Region, but only those who originated from and were financed from within the Health Region.

Ethical constraints

The study was given ethical approval on the understanding that any initial contact with people with PWS initiated by the research team, was made through a third party, in order to preserve confidentiality. This applied particularly to recruitment of people into the second phase, that is, the study of the PWS phenotype. For the prevalence study, ethical approval was given on the understanding that informants supplied only the initials, date of birth and gender of any people they knew who had been diagnosed with PWS or who fulfilled five or more of the criteria of the screening instrument described above. These informants were then asked to pass on letters from the Cambridge team to these nominees and their main carers, asking for their participation in the phenotypic study. Information sheets, a return form expressing interest or not, and a stamped, addressed envelope were enclosed. If a favourable response from the person with PWS, or suspected PWS, and their carer was received, the carer was contacted and a visit was arranged. This procedure applied to all group and professional nominees. Parents and carers who contacted the research team in response to media appeals were sent information packs directly.

The interviews

Interviews were conducted at a venue chosen by the participants, usually at their place of residence. One of the strengths of the project was that the same two researchers carried out all of the interviews throughout the project, and one of them performed all of the cognitive and attainment tests. This means that one possible source of variation in data collection – i.e. variation between interviewers or assessors – was not a problem. Travelling to and from these visits, and entering the data collected from the interviews and assessments into the computer database, gave the researchers the opportunity to discuss the information gained from the interviews and assessments. The three researchers based in Cambridge held frequent meetings at which any unusual or repeated observations and interview findings were reported. Impressions of both the person with PWS and the carer were discussed, comparisons were drawn between the current person and previously seen people and the published literature, and occasionally tentative hypotheses emerged that were then discussed with other team members.

Following introductions and general conversation with the person with PWS and the parent or other carer to establish rapport, the researchers outlined the project, answered questions and described the form of the interview and assessments, and the consent forms were then signed. At this time participants were asked if they were prepared to give a blood sample at a later date. One researcher then interviewed the informant while the other carried out the cognitive assessments and attainment tests.

The interviews were semi-structured, the interviewer reading out each question and, where appropriate, the interviewee was asked to elaborate on their answer – for example, to give a fuller description or an example to illustrate their answer. This format was also followed with the established questionnaires that formed part of the interview to the extent that questions, which the interviewee found ambiguous, were rephrased and elaborated answers were encouraged.

Research instruments

The first aim of the research project, which was to estimate the prevalence of PWS, required only a count of people with PWS. Since many people with a diagnosis of PWS had never had a genetic test, clinical diagnosis had to be accepted in the following situations: (1) where the person nominated as having PWS did not wish to take part in the project (31 nominations, of which eight came from genetics laboratories and therefore had a known genetic diagnosis); and (2) where a participant did not wish to provide a blood sample and had no previous genetic record (five people).

The second aim of the study, which was to describe the full range of the PWS phenotype, required a certain amount of selectivity of topics, because of time constraints. An important research instrument was a questionnaire compiled by the research group prior to the start of the project. The PWS Study Questionnaire comprised eight sections. Section One identified the person with PWS and the informant(s), usually a parent or main carer, by code numbers; the relationship of the informant to the person with PWS; and the date of birth, gestational age at birth, next of kin relationship and number of siblings of the person with PWS. Section Two asked about the presence or not of the clinical diagnostic criteria. Not all of the criteria were included. Notably, the question of dysmorphic features was omitted because, without objective measurements, it was considered to be too subjective. The informant's opinion was accepted as to the presence or not of a criterion, but the interviewer asked supplementary questions or asked for examples to clarify replies. For example, if the informant endorsed a high pain threshold, an example to illustrate this opinion was requested. Section Three asked about lifetime and recent eating behaviour; when access to food had to be controlled; how it was controlled, whether stealing and hoarding (of food or money) were problems;

and whether rotten food or non-food items had been eaten. There were also questions about fluid consumption, vomiting and constipation or diarrhoea. Section Four asked about behaviours associated with the syndrome: skin picking; temper tantrums; repetitive questioning; obsessional behaviour; violent or aggressive behaviour; mood fluctuations; argumentativeness; lying; stealing; stubbornness; and sense of humour. Section Five was devoted to general mental and physical health, including: anxiety; depression; heart problems; sleep apnoea; chest infections; scoliosis; diabetes mellitus; epilepsy; temperature regulation; noise tolerance; enuresis; and other problems. Section Six asked about lifetime medication: any regular medication; any growth hormone; and sex hormone treatments. This section also had a rough pain scale comprising the person's response to toothache, a broken bone, a trapped finger and a burn or scald. Section Seven asked about the person's childhood and included a screening for autistic traits, attention deficit and hyperactivity, as well as a record of schooling such as types of schools attended, ages at school changes and any problems at school. The final section asked about long-term illness or medical conditions in close family members and any unusual characteristics of the person with PWS. No questions were asked about family circumstances, socio-economic group or ethnicity. A copy of the questionnaire is included in an Appendix at the end of this chapter.

Direct assessments

Cognitive assessments used the Wechsler tests: Wechsler Pre-school and Primary Scale of Intelligence[1] (WPPSI) for 4- to 7-year-olds; Wechsler Intelligence Scale for Children[2] (WISC) for 8- to 16-year-olds; and Wechsler Adult Intelligence Scale[3] (WAIS) for 17-year-olds and above. In addition to providing a measure of overall IQ, these tests provide measures of the two major factors of IQ, verbal and visuo-spatial, and a profile of abilities measured by the various tests comprising the test battery. Tests used for educational attainments were the Wechsler Objective Reading Dimensions[4] (WORD), Wechsler Objective Language Dimensions[5] (WOLD) and Wechsler Objective Numerical Dimensions[6] (WOND) for ages 8 to 16 years and the Wide Range Achievement Test[7] (WRAT) for ages 17 years and over. The WORD-WOLD-WOND tests for the 8- to 16-year-olds cover reading, spelling, reading comprehension, receptive, expressive and written language, numerical operations and mathematics reasoning. The WRAT covers reading, spelling and arithmetic.

Informant questionnaires

The nature and extent of aberrant behaviour was measured using the Developmental Behaviour Checklist (DBC)[8] for children aged 4 to 17 years and by the Aberrant Behaviour Checklist (ABC)[9] for adults. Normative data for people with learning disabilities are available for these scales and for the subscales within them. The scales include questions about behaviours associated with PWS, such as temper tantrums, self injury (skin picking), mood swings and obsessional behaviour, and also questions relating to psychiatric symptoms, such as depression, withdrawal and anxiety.

The Vineland Adaptive Behaviour Scales[10], measuring levels of functioning in the three skill areas of communication, daily living and socialisation, were chosen because of their normalisation on groups of people with learning disabilities and because their frequent use in published research would make comparisons with other groups possible. The emphasis of the scales is not on what the person can do but what the person does do more or less routinely. The scales are not entirely suitable for people with PWS, since many questions are about food-related activities and, in the case of people with PWS, these activities may be restricted in order to prevent excessive eating.

The Life Experiences Checklist[11] measures opportunities enjoyed by the respondant in the areas of home, leisure, relationships, freedom and other opportunities. Mean score comparisons are available for a general population sample, broken down into urban, suburban and rural groups.

The Rutter Malaise Inventory[12] was administered to the parent or carer to get a measure of the stress caused by caring for a person with the syndrome. It was acknowledged that, in general, carers were not exclusively assigned to the person with PWS and that they were on duty only for a part of the time, whereas parents most often were the sole carers and had a full-time responsibility.

Disturbed or noisy sleep is one of the PWS diagnostic criteria and daytime sleepiness is a characteristic feature of the syndrome. For this reason the Maudsley Hospital Sleep Questionnaire[13] was chosen to measure these aspects of the phenotype. This instrument incorporates the Epworth Sleepiness Scale, which can be treated as an interval scale measure of daytime sleepiness.

Blood samples

Parents were initially asked for the results of previous genetic testing. However, it became apparent that few parents knew if and where genetic tests had been carried out, and even fewer parents knew the genetic subtype of their offspring. The latter finding meant that differences between genetic subtypes could not be investigated unless new genetic tests were undertaken. Blood samples were therefore requested from all participants willing to consent. Moreover, where consent was given, extracted RNA and DNA were stored to establish a resource for future research.

The procedure adopted was first to seek consent for a blood sample at the time of the assessment interview. (This meant that interviews and assessments of the participants took place blind to the genetic findings in most cases.) The participant's GP was then contacted and asked to take the blood sample as it was thought that having a familiar person take the sample would be more acceptable to participants. Alternatively, local hospitals were asked to undertake the venepuncture. Samples were then posted to the genetics laboratory. Where participants did not consent or it was not possible to obtain a blood sample, it was sometimes possible to obtain previous genetic records. This was done for 12 people, for six of whom the PWS genetic subtype was also recorded. There were eventually only five participants for whom there was neither a blood sample nor a previous record. All five had a previous clinical diagnosis.

Genetic procedures

For each of the blood samples received, DNA and RNA were extracted. Methylation analysis was undertaken at the *SNURF/SNRPN* locus and a genetic diagnosis of PWS confirmed only if a maternal band was detected.[14] Cytogenetic analysis was used to establish whether a deletion was present and parental samples were requested to confirm disomies. Microsatellite analysis at 10 or more loci spanning the entire deletion region from D15S11 to D15S219 was also undertaken.

Comparison groups

Parents and carers who responded to media appeals contacted the team directly by telephone. A few questions pertaining to the presence or not of clinical diagnostic criteria were sufficient to rule out some nominees as possible PWS, but some opted to join the study as part of a learning disabled control group. Others met the screening criteria and joined the group of people with possible PWS.

The criteria for the first comparison group were the presence of learning disabilities and being negative for the diagnosis of PWS. Most of the members of this comparison group were recruited through local schools for learning disabled children and care homes for adults with learning disabilities. Members recruited in this way were not asked to provide blood samples; otherwise they were treated similarly to the PWS participants. This comparison group was later augmented by those PWS nominees who gave a blood sample and were negative on the genetic tests and whose total score of the full range of diagnostic criteria was below our criterion.

A second comparison group was formed from those PWS nominees who gave a blood sample and were negative on the genetic tests and who also had missing data for the questions relating to the clinical diagnostic criteria (for example, birth and early infancy data was often missing in cases where parents were dead or the person was adopted) or whose total score was above our criterion. This group was analogous to those people referred to in the literature as PWS-like.

Augmenting the sample of people with PWS

As the population study progressed, it became clear that the number of people identified who had the disomy form of PWS would be too small for reliable statistical comparisons between genetic subgroups. The research team therefore recruited additional volunteers from outside the Anglia & Oxford Region, with preference given to those who were thought to have the disomy form of PWS, and to the residents in the PWS homes who were financed from outside the region.

Questions to be addressed by the Cambridge study

The identification, as described above, of as complete a group as possible of people with genetically confirmed PWS living in one region enables several important questions to be addressed that are best answered using such a population cohort. These are listed below and are covered in subsequent chapters:

1. Now that standard genetic tests are available that can reliably confirm the genetic diagnosis in over 99% of cases what is the true birth incidence and prevalence of PWS, and what is the age-related mortality rate? (Chapter 4.)
2. Which of the clinical criteria best predict a PWS genotype and how common are each of the clinical criteria in the PWS population? (Chapter 5.)
3. What is the distribution of IQ scores in the PWS population, what are their cognitive strengths and weaknesses, and is attainment in the basic skills of reading, spelling and arithmetic related to measured IQ in the same way as in the normal population or as in the learning disabled population? (Chapter 7.)
4. When compared to an IQ matched comparison group, does PWS have a distinct behavioural phenotype and, if so, what are the main characteristics of that phenotype, and what mechanisms might account for these behaviours? (Chapter 8.)
5. What medical conditions affect people with PWS, how frequently do they occur, and to what extent are they related to the obesity? (Chapter 9.)
6. Are rates of psychiatric illness in PWS the same as in the normal population or as in the learning disabled population? (Chapter 10.)
7. To what extent are people with PWS more obsessive than other learning disabled people and how is any obsessive behaviour best conceptualised? (Chapter 11.)
8. Are there cognitive, functional, or behavioural differences between the two main genetic subtypes of PWS and, if so, what mechanisms might account for these differences? (Chapters 6, 7, 10.)

Summary

Reasons for the Cambridge PWS population study:

1. To establish estimates for prevalence of people with genetically confirmed PWS.
2. To examine the age structure of people with PWS in the population.
3. To obtain a more representative sample of people with PWS for phenotypic studies.
4. To compare genetic and clinical findings in people with PWS.

Appendix 3.1

Contacts with groups and professionals in search for people with PWS

PWSA (UK).

Genetics Departments – all known post holders.

Paediatricians – registered members of the Royal College of Paediatricians.

Paediatricians – listed in the Anglia & Oxford Health Region Handbook.

Psychiatrists in learning disabilities – registered members of the Royal College of Psychiatrists.

Psychiatrists in learning disabilities – listed in the Anglia & Oxford Health Region Handbook.

General Practitioners – Cambridge area only (not cost effective).

Dieticians.

Community nurses.

County Councils – Special Education;
                                    – Social Services.

Special schools for learning disabilities.

Residential homes for learning disabilities.

Media – newspapers, television, radio.

Information given to contacts

Do you know anyone who has been diagnosed as having PWS or may have had **five** of the following characteristics:

Floppiness at birth

Initial failure to thrive or difficulty in sucking

The development of severe over-eating and rapid weight gain in early childhood

Obesity or the need for weight control

Problems with sexual development (e.g., undescended testes, delayed periods)

Some learning disability (mental handicap)

Small hands and feet

Short stature or the need for growth hormone

An abnormality of chromosome 15

The Prader–Willi Syndrome Study

Section 1

Personal information

Date of interview . . . .

Code number of person with PWS . . . .

Code number of informant 1 . . . .

Code number of informant 2 . . . .

Family/professional relationship to person with PWS. . . . .

Family/professional relationship to person with PWS. . . . .

Date of birth of person with PWS . . . .

Gestational age at birth (if known) . . . .

Next of kin (relationship) . . . .

Number of siblings (if known) . . . .

The Prader–Willi Syndrome Study

Section 2

Diagnostic Criteria

Were/are any of the following present:

1. Severe floppiness at birth with later improvement:	Yes	No	Don't know
2. Poor suck at birth with later improvement:	Yes	No	Don't know
3. Difficulty feeding at birth:	Yes	No	Don't know
4. Decreased movement of baby during pregnancy:	Yes	No	Don't know
5. Weak cry or inactivity as a baby:	Yes	No	Don't know
6. Obesity during childhood:	Yes	No	Don't know
If yes, at what age did this first develop:	. . . .	years	
what has been his/her maximum weight:	. . . .	Kgms	. . . . . sto/lbs
at what age was this weight reached:	. . . .	years	
7. Tendency to overeat or obsession with food:	Yes	No	Don't know
If yes, at what age was this first noticed:	. . . .	years	
8. *For males:*			
Undescended testes:	Yes	No	Don't know
Surgery on testes:	Yes	No	Don't know

If yes, were any testes actually removed:	None	One	Both
Decreased facial and body hair:	Yes	No	Don't know
Lack of voice change:	Yes	No	Don't know
At what age did voice change:	. . . .	years	

For females:

Does/did she have periods: (say no if they only occurred while on the pill)	Yes	No	Don't know
If yes, when did she have her first period:	. . . .	years	
how many times a year did she have periods (not on pill)	times/year		
9. Learning difficulties:	Yes	No	Don't know
10. Disturbed or noisy sleep:	Yes	No	Don't know
11. Short height:	Yes	No	Don't know
Centile	. . . .		
What is his/her height:	. . . .	metres	. . . . . ft/ins
How tall is his/her mother:	. . .	metres	. . . . . ft/ins
How tall is his/her father:	. . . .	metres	. . . . . ft/ins
12. Fair skin and hair compared with family:	Yes	No	Don't know
13. Small hands or feet:	Yes	No	Don't know
14. Eye problems:	Yes	No	Don't know
short sight:	Yes	No	Don't know
squint:	Yes	No	Don't know
15. Thick saliva with crusting at corners of mouth:	Yes	No	Don't know
16. Difficulty with articulating words:	Yes	No	Don't know
17. High pain threshold:	Yes	No	Don't know
18. Not feeling hot or cold when others are:	Yes	No	Don't know

19. Thin bones – for example easily broken:	Yes	No	Don't know
If yes, give example:	. . . .		
20. Unusual skill with jigsaws:	Yes	No	Don't know
21. Has genetic testing been done:	Yes	No	Don't know
If yes, result, if known:	. . . .		
Where was the testing done:	. . . .		
(Ask if willing to have another test for our use)	Yes	No	Don't know

The Prader–Willi Syndrome Study

Section 3

Eating Behaviour

Lifetime eating behaviour (N/A = Infant, no problems as yet)

These questions refer to eating behaviour over the lifetime of the person with PWS (i.e. from when the eating problems were first noticed).

Over what proportion of his/her lifetime has it been necessary to control access to food?

Not at all . . . .
Less than half . . . .
Approximately half . . . .
More than half . . . .
All . . . .

Over his/her lifetime what has been the most common method you have used to try to control his/her weight?

None have been necessary . . . .
Reminders about diet only . . . .
Supervision at meal times only . . . .
Supervised access to food at all times . . . .
Supervised access, locking of cupboards, etc . . . .

Over what proportion of his/her lifetime has he/she engaged in the following behaviours:

1. Stealing food or stealing money to buy food:

   Not at all . . . .
   Less than half . . . .
   Approximately half . . . .
   More than half . . . .
   All . . . .

2. Hoarding food or objects:
   Not at all . . . .
   Less than half . . . .
   Approximately half . . . .
   More than half . . . .
   All . . . .
3. Eating rotten food or normally inedible substances:
   Not at all . . . .
   Less than half . . . .
   Approximately half . . . .
   More than half . . . .
   All . . . .
   Give examples: . . . .

Recent eating behaviour

These questions refer to the eating behaviour of the person with PWS over the past few months. Over an average 28 days were rules necessary to control his/her eating behaviour?

Not at all . . . .
Less than half the days . . . .
Approximately half the days . . . .
More than half the days . . . .
Everyday . . . .

If rules were necessary, what was the main method used to try to control his/her eating behaviour and weight over an average 28 days?

None have been necessary . . . .
Reminders about diet only . . . .
Supervision at meal times only . . . .
Supervised access to food at all times . . . .
Supervised access, locking of cupboards, etc . . . .

Over an average 28 days did he/she break the rules?

Not at all . . . .
Less than half the days . . . .
Approximately half the days . . . .
More than half the days . . . .
Everyday . . . .

Fluid Consumption

These questions refer to the amount of fluids consumed by the person with PWS.
How much fluid is drunk by the person with PWS in an average day?

0 to 3 cups . . . .
4 to 10 cups . . . .
10 to 15 cups . . . .
16 to 20 cups . . . .
More than 20 cups . . . .

Has the amount of fluid drunk in an average day ever changed noticeably?

Yes . . . .
No . . . .
Don't know . . . .

If so, was the change associated with other changes in behaviour or health?

Eating behaviour . . . .
Medication . . . .
Exercise . . . .
Diabetes . . . .
Other . . . .

Please give details: . . . .

Vomiting

These questions refer to vomiting behaviour of the person with PWS.

Has he/she ever been known to vomit?   Yes   No   Don't know
Or regurgitate?
   If yes, how often has this occurred on average: . . . . . . times per year

   Under what circumstances: . . . .

Constipation

Does he/she regularly suffer from constipation?   Yes   No   Don't know
Or diarrhoea?

Does this require treatment?   Yes   No   Don't know

The Prader–Willi Syndrome Study

Other Behaviours

These questions refer to the presence or not of other behaviour problems and their severity.

0 = never been a problem
1 = a problem but only for a brief period
2 = continuous minor problem (less than once a week)
3 = can be severe (at least weekly) but intermittent
4 = severe problem occurring more than once a week
7 = age appropriate only
8 = not applicable

	Ever	In the past month
Skin picking	. . . .	. . . .
Temper tantrums	. . . .	. . . .
Repetitive questioning	. . . .	. . . .
Obsessional behaviour	. . . .	. . . .
Violent/aggressive b'h'r	. . . .	. . . .
Fluctuations in mood	. . . .	. . . .
Tendency to argue	. . . .	. . . .
Lying	. . . .	. . . .
Stealing	. . . .	. . . .
Other b'h'r problem	. . . .	. . . .

Explain . . . .

Stubborn to unusual degree . . . .
Sense of humour? . . . .
Nature of humour . . . .

The Prader–Willi Syndrome Study

Section 5

General Health

These questions refer to the general health of the person with PWS during their lifetime.

Has he/she ever had the following health problems and, if so has he/she received treatment for the problem:

Severe anxiety lasting more than a few days:	Yes	No	Don't know
Age of first onset:	. . . .	years	
Treatment received	Yes	No	Don't know
Severe depression lasting more than a few days:	Yes	No	Don't know
Age of first onset:	. . . .	years	
Treatment received	Yes	No	Don't know
Any other nervous problem lasting more than a few days:	Yes	No	Don't know
Age of first onset:	. . . .	years	
Treatment received	Yes	No	Don't know
Heart problems:	Yes	No	Don't know
Age of first onset:	. . . .	years	
Treatment received	Yes	No	Don't know
Sleep apnoea (disturbed and noisy sleep):	Yes	No	Don't know
Age of first onset:	. . . .	years	
Treatment received	Yes	No	Don't know
Recurrent chest infections:	Yes	No	Don't know

Age of first onset:	. . . .	years	
Treatment received	Yes	No	Don't know
Scoliosis (curvature of the spine):	Yes	No	Don't know
Age of first onset:	. . . .	years	
Treatment received	Yes	No	Don't know
Diabetes mellitus (sugar diabetes):	Yes	No	Don't know
Age of first onset:	. . . .	years	
Treatment received	Yes	No	Don't know
Medication (say what)			
When medication started	. . . .	years	
Any complications of diabetes	Yes	No	Don't know
(details and age of onset)			
Epilepsy/fits/attacks of dizziness:	Yes	No	Don't know
Age of first onset:	. . . .	years	
Treatment received	Yes	No	Don't know
Description of attacks:.			
Abnormal temperature (shivering, sweating):	Yes	No	Don't know
Age of first onset:	. . . .	years	
Treatment received	Yes	No	Don't know
Abnormal noise tolerance/intolerance:	Yes	No	Don't know
Age of first onset:	. . . .	years	
Treatment received	Yes	No	Don't know
Enuresis (bed wetting):	Yes	No	Don't know
Age of first onset:	. . . .	years	
Treatment received	Yes	No	Don't know
Others (please specify below):	Yes	No	Don't know
Age of first onset:	. . . .	years	
Treatment received	Yes	No	Don't know
Specification:			

The Prader–Willi Syndrome Study

Medication

Please list any medication he/she has received regularly (including hormone replacement):

Name of medication:	. . . .	. . . .
Dose:	. . . .	. . . .
Age when first started:	. . . .	. . . .
What is it for:	. . . .	. . . .
Effectiveness:	. . . .	. . . .
Name of medication:	. . . .	. . . .
Dose:	. . . .	. . . .
Age when first started:	. . . .	. . . .
What is it for:	. . . .	. . . .
Effectiveness:	. . . .	. . . .
Name of medication:	. . . .	. . . .
Dose:	. . . .	. . . .
Age when first started:	. . . .	. . . .
What is it for:	. . . .	. . . .
Effectiveness:	. . . .	. . . .

Has he/she ever received growth hormone treatment?   Yes   No   Don't know

If yes, between which ages: . . . . years   . . . . years

Were there any associated changes in b'h'r?   Yes   No   Don't know

What were these changes?   . . . .

Has he/she ever received sex hormone treatment?	Yes	No	Don't know

If yes, between which ages: . . . . years . . . . . . years

What hormones were given: . . . .

Were there any associated changes in b'h'r?	Yes	No	Don't know

What were these changes . . . .

Pain

Does he/she have an unusual response to painful stimuli: Marked mild/no/don't know

Has he/she ever used pain killers?	Yes		No	Don't know

If yes, were they: Bought over the counter Prescribed by a doctor Given in hospital

Why were they taken . . . .

Has he/she ever had:	toothache	broken bone	trapped finger	burn/scald
Did he/she show pain:	. . . .	. . . .	. . . .	. . . .
Were pain killers used:	. . . .	. . . .	. . . .	. . . .

The Prader–Willi Syndrome Study

Section 7

Childhood

These questions refer to the childhood of the person with PWS.

As a young child, is/was he/she more withdrawn or more out-going?   withdrawn   out-going

Examples: . . . .

Does/did he/she show any of the following to an unusual degree:

Makes careless mistakes:	Yes	No	Don't know	From/to . . . . .years
Difficulty sustaining attention:	Yes	No	Don't know	From/to . . . . .years
Does not seem to listen when spoken to directly	Yes	No	Don't know	From/to . . . . .years
Fails to follow simple instructions/finish tasks (not due to opposition or understanding)	Yes	No	Don't know	From/to . . . . .years
Difficulty organising tasks/activity	Yes	No	Don't know	From/to . . . . .years
Avoids sustained mental effort	Yes	No	Don't know	From/to . . . . .years
Often loses tools/equipment	Yes	No	Don't know	From/to . . . . .years
Is often distracted by extraneous stimuli	Yes	No	Don't know	From/to . . . . .years

Is often forgetful in daily activities	Yes	No	Don't know	From/to . . . . .years
Often fidgets with hands or feet	Yes	No	Don't know	From/to . . . . .years
Often leaves seat	Yes	No	Don't know	From/to . . . . .years
Often runs about or climbs in inappropriate situations	Yes	No	Don't know	From/to . . . . .years
Has difficulty playing quietly	Yes	No	Don't know	From/to . . . . .years
Is always 'on the go'	Yes	No	Don't know	From/to . . . . .years
Often talks excessively	Yes	No	Don't know	From/to . . . . .years
Often blurts out answers before questions completed	Yes	No	Don't know	From/to . . . . .years
Has difficulty awaiting turn	Yes	No	Don't know	From/to . . . . .years
Often interrupts/intrudes on others	Yes	No	Don't know	From/to . . . . .years

Does/did he/she show any of the following to an unusual degree:

Hardly ever initiates(d) conversation	Yes	No	Don't know	From/to . . . . .years
Frequently indulges(d) in repetitive talk	Yes	No	Don't know	From/to . . . . .years
Shows(ed) very little emotional expression	Yes	No	Don't know	From/to . . . . .years
Hardly ever calls(ed) attention to things (4–5 yrs)	Yes	No	Don't know	From/to . . . . .years
Hardly ever smiles(d) in response (4–5 yrs)	Yes	No	Don't know	From/to . . . . .years
Hardly ever indulges(d) in co-operative play (4–5 yrs)	Yes	No	Don't know	From/to . . . . .years
Hardly ever makes(made) eye-contact (4–5 yrs)	Yes	No	Don't know	From/to . . . . .years
Hardly ever indulges in imaginative play (4–5 yrs)	Yes	No	Don't know	From/to . . . . .years

Schooling

Has he/she ever had any formal schooling (any type):	Yes	No	Don't know
Did he/she ever attend playgroup or nursery school:	Yes	No	Don't know

    If yes, between what ages: . . . . years to . . . . . . .years

    Were there any special difficulties: Yes   No   Don't know

    If yes, what were they:

    . . . .

  Did he/she ever attend a special school: Yes   No   Don't know

    If yes, between what ages: . . . . .years to . . . . . . .years

    Were there any special difficulties: Yes   No   Don't know

    If yes, what were they:

    . . . .

  Did he/she ever attend infant school: Yes   No   Don't know

    If yes, between what ages: . . . . .years to . . . . . . .years

    Were there any special difficulties: Yes   No   Don't know

    If yes, what were they:

    . . . .

  Did he/she ever attend junior school: Yes   No   Don't know

    If yes, between what ages: . . . . .years to . . . . . . .years

    Were there any special difficulties: Yes   No   Don't know

    If yes, what were they:

    . . . .

  Did he/she ever attend secondary school: Yes   No   Don't know

    If yes, between what ages: . . . . .years to . . . . . . .years

    Were there any special difficulties: Yes   No   Don't know

    If yes, what were they:

    . . . .

  Has he/she ever taken an ability or IQ test: Yes   No   Don't know

    If yes, what was his/her IQ   . . . .

The Prader–Willi Syndrome Study

Section 8

Comments

Has any close family member (sibling, parent, grandparent) of x got a disability, long-term illness or other medical condition?

Is there anything else unusual about x?

Thank you very much for answering these questions. If you have any other comments you would like to make, please do so.

REFERENCES

1. Wechsler, D. *Pre-school and Primary Scale of Intelligence (WPPSI-Revised UK)*. Psychological Corporation. London: Harcourt Brace & Co. 1993.
2. Wechsler, D. *Wechsler Intelligence Scale for Children (WISCIII – UK)*. Psychological Corporation. London: Harcourt Brace & Co. 1993.
3. Wechsler, D. *The Wechsler Adult Intelligence Scale (WAIS-Revised* UK Edition). Psychological Corporation. London: Harcourt Brace & Co. 1993.
4. Wechsler, D. *Wechsler Objective Reading Dimensions (WORD)*. Psychological Corporation. London: Harcourt Brace & Co. 1993.
5. Rust, J. *Wechsler Objective Language Dimensions (WOLD)*. Psychological Corporation. London: Harcourt Brace & Co. 1995.
6. Rust, J. *Wechsler Objective Numerical Dimensions (WOND)*. Psychological Corporation. London: Harcourt Brace & Co. 1995.
7. Wilkinson, G. S. *The Wide Range Achievement Test (WRAT-3)*. Psychological Corporation. London: Harcourt Brace & Co. 1993.
8. Einfeld, S. & Tonge, B. J. *Developmental Behaviour Checklist – Parental Version*. Clayton, Australia: Centre for Developmental Psychiatry, 1989.
9. Aman, M. G., Singh, N. N., Stewart, A. W. *et al. Aberrant Behavior Checklist*. New York: Slosson, 1986.
10. Sparrow, S. S., Balla, D. A. & Cicchetti, D. V. *Vineland Adaptive Behavior Scales*. Windsor: NFER-Nelson, 1984.
11. Ager, A. *Life Experiences Checklist*. Windsor: NFER-Nelson, 1990.
12. Rutter, M. Malaise inventory. In Rutter, M., Tizard, J. & Kingsley Whitmore, K. (Eds). *Education, Health and Behaviour*. Appendix 7. London: Longman, 1981.
13. Johns, M. W. A new method for measuring daytime sleepiness: the Epworth Sleepiness Scale. *Sleep* **14** (1991), 540–545.
14. American Society of Human Genetics/American College of Medical Genetics Test and Technology Transfer Committee. Diagnostic testing for Prader–Willi and Angelman syndromes: report of the ASHG/ACMG Test and Technology Transfer Committee. *American Journal of Human Genetics* **58** (1996), 1085–1088.

Part II

Prader–Willi syndrome prevalence, phenotypic functioning and characteristics

4

Prevalence, birth incidence and mortality

Previous population studies

In the literature on PWS, prevalence has been variously quoted as 'about 1 in 25,000 live births',[1] 'between one in 25,000 and one in 10,000 live born children',[2] '[estimates] vary 6-fold from 1 in 5,000 to 10,000; 1 in 10,000; 1 in 15,000; 1 in 25,000; to 1 in 10,000 to 30,000'.[3] These estimates are confusing because some authors use the term prevalence where others use birth incidence. We use birth incidence to refer to the number of live births of babies with PWS and prevalence to refer to the number of people with PWS of all ages in the population. Only two estimates appear to be based on epidemiological data, those of Akefeldt et al.[2] and Burd et al.[3] (see Chapter 1). In the North Dakota study (Burd et al.[3]) the authors used similar informants to those contacted in the Cambridge study. The ascertainment methods used in the North Dakota study identified eight males, eight females and one person whose gender was not given, with an age range from 9 to 30 years. At that time the population of North Dakota for that age range was 263 444, giving a prevalence rate of 1:16 062, equivalent to 1:38 395 in the entire population. No figures were given for the number of people with a genetic diagnosis, and the diagnostic assessment was based, in at least some cases, on a one-page questionnaire pictorially demonstrating the signs of PWS to aid identification. Birth incidence was not estimated.

In the Akefeldt study in the rural Swedish county of Skaraborg only the prevalence of PWS in the age range 0 to 25 years was estimated. The methods were again similar to those of the Cambridge study, including the use of selected diagnostic criteria for PWS to identify possible cases. However, the study did not use genetic tests to confirm PWS, but instead, clinical diagnoses were made on the basis of the findings of a neuropaediatrician, a child psychiatrist, a child psychologist and a speech pathologist. Eleven people (seven male and four female) were considered to definitely have PWS and a further five (two male and three female) were considered probable. These numbers gave a population prevalence of 'clear PWS' up to age 25 years of 1:8500, and between 7 and 25 years, 1:8000. If the people with suspected PWS were also included, these prevalence rates became 1:6700 and 1:5000, respectively. The diagnosis was confirmed genetically in only five people, all of whom had chromosome 15 deletions. Birth incidence was not estimated.

These different population estimates can be reconciled in several ways, including the different clinical criteria used for diagnosis, sampling errors, high mortality rates between the ages of 25 and 30, or varying prevalence rates in different populations. The two studies certainly used different criteria. The Burd *et al.* study used five drawings illustrating their criteria with the instruction 'Please check that all are present in your patient'. The criteria corresponding to the drawings were: hypotonia; poor suck; early history of feeding problems; small hands and feet; hyperphagia after the first year with obesity; bitemporal narrowing of the head; prominent forehead; strabismus; dysplastic ears; narrow external canal; triangular upper lip; fat face with micrognathia; short stature; decreased muscle with increased adipose tissue; atrophic scrotum; and small testes and penis. The Akefeldt *et al.* study had the criteria of severe hypotonia in the neonatal period, hypogonadism/delayed sexual development, major weight problems and learning disorder, and the supportive criteria of a deletion of chromosome 15, short stature, typical dysmorphic features, typical personality traits, scoliosis and skin picking.

When considering the possible sources of error in these two studies, experience from the Cambridge Study, which combined the use of genetic and clinical criteria, suggested that both of these earlier studies probably included people who would have been found not to have PWS if they had been investigated genetically. High mortality rates in PWS have never been reported as specific to a particular age group, but intuitively it would seem a possible explanation for the difference in prevalence rates, given that the Swedish study was of a younger population. This has been examined further in the Cambridge study. The final possible explanation, that there might be differing prevalence rates in different populations, is at odds with the accepted view of PWS as a randomly occurring *de novo* genetic fault. This accepted view is supported by the fact that in both studies the gender ratio is close to 1:1, if, in the Swedish study, people with 'probable' as well as 'definite' PWS are included. Clearly, if the true explanation is that prevalence rates vary depending on the population studied, then these estimates cannot be generalised to other countries. In the Cambridge study, the aim was to sample a larger population base so that more accurate estimates of birth incidence and age-related prevalence could be obtained, and comparisons could be made within the population sample in order to identify whether differences in prevalence across populations and ages were true, or a result of age-specific mortality or sampling bias.

The Cambridge PWS population study

The Cambridge population prevalence study in the UK was undertaken in the old Anglia & Oxford Health Region (see Chapter 3). All ages were included, so as to obtain some estimate of mortality rates in the PWS population, and as far as possible the diagnosis was made by the routine diagnostic method using *SNRPN* methylation[4] or, if that was not possible, the presence of accepted diagnostic criteria.

Since the ideal method of random sampling is impractical for rare disorders that require clinical diagnosis, the method of counting all known cases in the region was used, as it was in the studies quoted above. The size of the region studied was chosen after administrative and statistical considerations. The region chosen comprises approximately five million people – about one-tenth of the population of England and Wales. The population prevalence rates found in the previous studies quoted above, together with statistical power considerations, suggested that the study of the phenotype would require a population of at least this size.

Health, education and social services professionals were contacted and sent a list of common PWS characteristics and asked if they knew of anyone fulfilling at least half of these (see Chapter 3 Appendix). In addition, the UK PWS Association was asked to advise about numbers known to the Association living in the study area. To preserve anonymity, initials, gender and date of birth (or age) of their nominees were requested. These were necessary in order to avoid double counting of people who possibly had the syndrome. Anonymity and indirect contact were conditions of ethical approval for the study. Therefore no other details of people nominated who did not agree to participate further are available. All responders who were willing were recruited into the phenotypic study for cognitive assessment of the person with PWS and in-depth interviews (including a section asking about the presence or not of the symptoms included in the consensus diagnostic criteria) with a parent or main carer or both. Blood samples were later collected from all those who were willing and able to provide samples. When the participant was unwilling or there were difficulties obtaining a sample, permission was sought for access to previous genetic records. For most participants in the phenotypic study, therefore, a diagnosis of PWS could be confirmed either clinically (parents/carers were asked at interview about the presence or not of consensus diagnostic criteria) and/or genetically. In the region there is a collection of group homes for people with PWS. Only those funded from within the study region were included in the population study, the people funded from outside the region were excluded from this part of the study.

Prevalence

During the active period of the study (between September 1998 and June 2000) 167 people with a diagnosis of PWS or with PWS symptoms were notified to us from the sources listed earlier, including nominations by parents and other relatives of people with eating problems and other PWS symptoms, who responded to media appeals. Figure 4.1 shows the breakdown of this group in terms of participation in the phenotypic study, blood samples obtained, genetic test results and clinical diagnoses. This figure shows that after eliminating those nominees who were found to have died, were untraceable, found on preliminary investigation not to have PWS or had moved out of the region, 123 people with possible PWS were included. Of these 123, thirty-one with a previous diagnosis of PWS did not wish to participate in the phenotypic study, and therefore the only data pertaining to them was that provided by those who referred the person to the research study. Eight of these 31 individuals were nominated by genetics laboratories, and for the remaining 23 individuals the genetic status was not given. Of the 123 nominees, 75 were from multiple sources, as detailed in Table 4.1. Many were nominated as 'maybe', particularly parental nominations. None of the 31 not seen were classified 'maybe'. Table 4.1 also gives the number of people seen who were positive for PWS against the total number seen from the various sources.

Among the 92 who agreed in principle to participate in the phenotypic study, genetic testing was possible with 67 participants. Of the other 25, eight were considered not to have PWS at interview. For another 12, results of previous genetic tests were obtained which confirmed the diagnoses. The remaining five for whom no blood sample was obtained were included as they met clinical criteria. One of these people was later confirmed genetically as having PWS on methylation analysis using DNA obtained from a buccal smear. Altogether, 27 people out of 92 were deemed not to have PWS (the above eight on clinical grounds only, 11 on both clinical and genetic grounds, a further eight on genetic grounds) and 65 met clinical and/or genetic criteria. Our incidence and prevalence report was based on the latter group (65 people) and the 31 who did not wish to be involved in the larger study (where records strongly supported the diagnosis), giving a total of 96 people who the researchers were fully confident had PWS. Figure 4.2 shows the frequencies by age (standardised to midnight 31.12.99) of these 96 people.

There were two obvious potential sources of error in our results: false positives (people considered to have PWS but who do not) and missing cases (people in the population with PWS but who were not identified). With respect to the former,

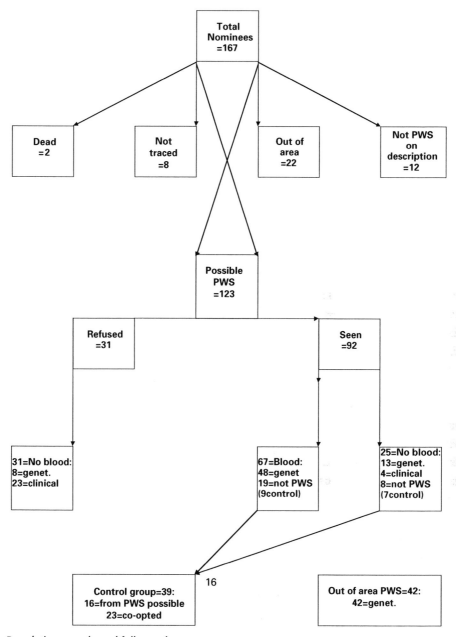

Figure 4.1.   Population sample and full sample.

Table 4.1. Population classification of Prader–Willi syndrome (PWS) nominees by source

	Genetic diagnosis PWS	Clinical diagnosis PWS	Not seen	Non-PWS	%positive of those seen
Genetics laboratory	32	0	8	0	100
Doctors	87	5	23	15	86
PWSA (UK)	36	1	13	10	79
Relative	6	0	1	13	32
Head teacher	8	0	2	0	100
Social Services	10	1	3	2	85
Home/centre manager	1	0	0	1	50

among those people seen, we had 60 people with genetic confirmation and five who did not have a genetic test (three refused, two tried and failed) but who met clinical diagnostic criteria. Among the 31 not seen, eight had genetic confirmation. The findings summarised in Table 4.1 suggested that at least 80% of the others were expected to be positive, so that we anticipated that at most there would only be five people who were false positives, and even fewer when the firmness of the nominations was considered.

With respect to missing cases, we believed this to be more problematic for several reasons. The weakest evidence for missing cases is regional variation in prevalence; much stronger evidence was age by county and gender variations. Table 4.2 gives the numbers of people with PWS divided according to each county. The overall population rate was 1:52 000, with county rates varying from 1:42 000 to 1:67 000 (not statistically significant). This could have indicated that identification was better in some areas than in others, and a conservative estimate suggested that there may have been another seven people with PWS within those counties that reported low rates. However, this variation may also have been random.

Table 4.3 gives the numbers of people with probable or definite PWS across the age range. Assuming that roughly the same number of babies with PWS are born every year, an examination of the overall age structure of our sample suggests that some very young children with PWS may not have been diagnosed (see Table 4.3), awaiting the onset of eating and behaviour problems to prompt later investigations. (This is supported by age at diagnosis data collected in interviews; new diagnoses were common in the first year and again between three and five years.) If we assume a zero mortality rate for children under six years, Table 4.3 suggests that as many as five children with PWS were not yet diagnosed. The age structure of identified cases within counties also supported the 'missing cases' hypothesis. In Norfolk, for example, only one person was under 18 years out of 13 identified, while in Berkshire there was only one person with PWS over 17 years out of 11 identified.

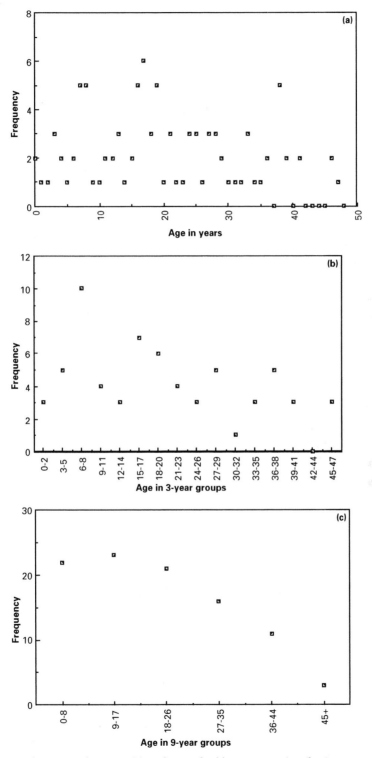

Figure 4.2.   Age frequency data, raw (a) and smoothed by age grouping (b, c).

Table 4.2. Numbers, gender differences and ages of people with Prader–Willi syndrome identified by county

	Beds	Berks	Bucks	Cambs	Norfolk	N'thants	Oxon	Suffolk
Male	7	4	7	10	9	6	5	7
Female	4	6	6	3	3	2	4	5
Not stated	–	1	2	1	1	3	–	–
Totals	11	11	15	14	13	11	9	12
Age in years								
0–2	–	2	1	–	–	–	–	1
3–5	–	–	2	3	1	–	–	–
6–8	2	4	2	3	–	–	1	–
9–11	–	1	1	1	–	–	–	1
12–14	1	1	2	1	–	–	1	–
15–17	–	2	2	3	–	2	2	2
18–20	1	–	1	1	3	1	–	2
21–23	1	–	–	–	3	–	–	1
24–26	2	–	1	–	–	1	3	–
27–29	1	–	1	1	1	3	–	1
30–32	–	–	1	–	1	–	1	–
33–35	1	–	–	–	–	2	–	2
36–38	1	1	1	1	1	–	1	1
39–41	–	–	–	–	3	1	–	–
42–44	–	–	–	–	–	–	–	–
45–47	1	–	–	–	–	1	–	1

In all but one county, we found more males than females (55 male, 33 female, eight gender not stated). Assuming that the gender ratio in PWS is close to unity as the two previous studies[2,3] found, it therefore appeared that females with PWS were either specifically not diagnosed or had been less likely to be referred to the study than males. We estimated that there may have been between 14 and 30 more females with PWS in the region. Of the four infants aged 0–2 years, three were male, and in both Cambridgeshire and Norfolk we found six more males than females (see Table 4.2).

Estimated population prevalence, birth incidence and age-specific mortality rate

As stated above, the overall prevalence rate was found to be 1:52 000. Unlike the previous population studies, which yielded 17 probable people with PWS (age

Table 4.3. Numbers across the former Anglia &
Oxford Health Region divided by age and sex

Age (years)	Male	Female	Not stated	Total
0–2	3	1	–	4
3–5	3	2	1	6
6–8	5	6	1	12
9–11	3	1	–	4
12–14	3	3	–	6
15–17	6	6	1	13
18–20	7	2	–	9
21–23	4	1	–	5
24–26	6	1	–	7
27–29	6	1	1	8
30–32	1	1	1	3
33–35	1	3	1	5
36–38	3	3	1	7
39–41	3	0	1	4
42–44	0	0	–	0
45–47	1	2	–	3
Total	55	33	8	96

range 9–30 years) in North Dakota, and 16 people with PWS (age 0–25 years) in
Skaraborg, we had a sufficiently large sample to look at age-specific prevalences.
A number of different methods were available to estimate birth incidence from
the raw data (Figure 4.2a). All methods depended on the different assumptions we
were prepared to make. The chief assumption was that PWS is due to a randomly-
occurring genetic fault and that the age frequencies constitute a random sequence
about a steady incidence rate. (We note that this sequence would vary slightly if we
had chosen a different date for age standardisation.) This sequence was smoothed
in various ways, as shown in Figure 4.2, where the data were grouped in three-year
and in nine-year intervals. In the latter case, the data were fit by a quadratic with
an $R^2 = 0.996$ (an exceptionally good fit). We also assumed no false positives in
ascertainment. This then gives lower bounds for the prevalence, birth incidence,
and mortality rate, for a particular method of calculation (that is, a particular
method of grouping the data).

For example, assuming no missing data and using the smoothed data obtained
from the nine-year grouping, we found prevalence rates of 22, 23, 21 people with
PWS in the first three, nine-year periods, a rate of 1:28 000, with a zero mortality
rate to age 27 years and thereafter an average mortality rate of 6.1% (from 2.44

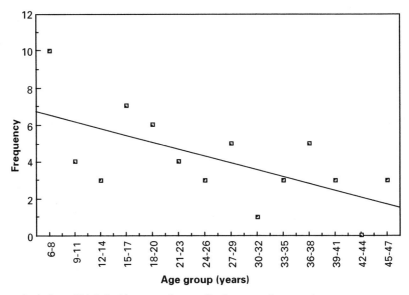

Figure 4.3.   Calculation of birth incidence and mortality from age frequencies.

to 0 in 20 years). A similar calculation (data not shown) with 8-year grouping (fit by a quadratic with $R^2 = 0.85$) and rates of 17, 17, 25, 17 people with PWS in the first four, eight-year periods, gave a rate of 1:29 000, with a zero rate of mortality to age 32 and thereafter an average mortality rate of 7.9% (from 2.375 to 0 in 15 years).

From the above this suggests that data are missing (females) but may be fairly evenly spread across the age groups (age by county). If this is the case, then the decrease in the number of people with PWS in older age groups is probably due to an increased mortality rate and we could use the whole distribution to estimate lower bounds for birth incidence and mortality rate. This was our preferred method of estimating these quantities. Figure 4.3 illustrates this method, where the fitted line is the result of ignoring ages 0–5 years (since we hypothesised that infants might be missing in this age range, their eventual diagnosis awaiting the onset of the second phase of PWS symptoms). A straight line, as shown, was found to be near the optimum fit with $R^2 = 0.41$ (R^2 could be increased to 0.44 by fitting a fourth order polynomial). This would imply a steady death rate across the age groups, rather than an increasing rate with age. (Anecdotally, we were told of two people with probable PWS who died before we could see them: a 3- to 4-year-old girl and a 13-year-old boy.) By extrapolation from Figure 4.3, we see that 10.2 children are expected in the age range 0–2 years (i.e. in 3 years), giving a birth incidence of 1:20 000 in the population studied (68 000 births per year). We also see that the overall death rate in this PWS population is about 3% per year (i.e. from 3.4 to zero over 56 years). This compares with an overall death rate in the population of England

and Wales of about 1% per year, and only about 0.13% per year in those up to 55 years.

Another possible hypothesis was that advances in genetics would result in increasing numbers of people identified and given an accurate diagnosis. If this had been the case, ascertainment by age would be a step function, with steps corresponding to identification of the genetic characteristics of PWS – i.e. chromosome 15 deletions (*c.* 1981, age 18 years), maternal chromosome 15 disomy (*c.* 1989, age 10 years) and the imprinting centre methylation tests (*c.* 1995, age 4 years). This particular hypothesis was not supported by our data.

A final hypothesis was that data were missing only, or mainly, from the older age groups. This is consistent with the eight-year and nine-year groupings, if we assume little or no mortality. But there are two arguments against this. First, the county data and age at diagnosis data suggested that missing people with PWS were not confined to older age groups. In some counties such age groups are over-represented. Second, several older people were nominated as possibly having PWS and were interviewed but were found to be genetically negative. So failure to find older people was not due to lack of candidates.

Discussion of the findings

There were a number of problems related to this method of conducting a prevalence study of PWS. The three main questions were: How should PWS be defined?; Do all nominees have PWS?; and Do all other people in the region *not* have PWS?

The first question regarding the definitive diagnosis to some extent remains unresolved as neither the genetic test nor the clinical diagnosis is 100% definitive. Although it is generally agreed that genetic abnormalities of the Prader–Willi critical region on the chromosome 15 of paternal origin underlie the clinical manifestations of the syndrome, and that the dual genetic tests used will probably detect 99% of such abnormalities, the precise gene(s) involved have not been identified, and therefore a definitive genetic test is not available. From the clinical perspective, it is clear that there are other chromosomal abnormalities, such as deletions of part of chromosome 6, that are associated with PWS-like symptoms (one such person is known to us), which demonstrated that reliance on clinical diagnosis may have resulted in the inclusion of those whose clinical phenotype results from a different genotype. There was one person in our population study with a score of 9 on the diagnostic criteria who was excluded when extensive genetic tests proved negative.

With respect to the answer to the second question, as to whether all nominees have PWS, we could not be certain. Some nominated did not respond to requests to take part in the phenotype study, and therefore we had to rely on previous clinical and/or genetic data. Others did not wish for a blood test and, in the absence of a previous test, a genetic diagnosis was not possible. However, we were restrictive about who was or was not included. We excluded all those 27 nominees who did not meet clinical criteria, genetic criteria, or both clinical and genetic criteria for PWS. These people had normal maternal and paternal methylation patterns and gene expression at the *SNRPN* locus (where blood was available) and typically had less than 50% of the required diagnostic criteria. We included 60 people who had definite genetic diagnoses and five others who had definite clinical diagnoses (in the absence of genetic confirmation). The 31 who did not wish to participate in the phenotypic study were all included as having PWS, as detailed earlier.

Our assessment of findings relevant to the third question (whether all others in the region do not have PWS) leads us to believe that there were other people in the region who do have PWS. If it is assumed that the syndrome is indeed caused solely by random genetic error (i.e. with no environmental component), it follows that prevalence should not be biased with respect to gender, race or environment. Although some relationship to paternal occupation in the hydrocarbon industry had been described in the past, which might possibly lead to clustering,[5] this finding has not been replicated. With the above assumptions, it was possible to look for internal consistencies within our regional sample, such as by county, by gender, or by race. There was not enough variation in racial background to test our sample with respect to race. In all but one county, we found more males than females (55 male, 33 female, eight gender not stated). This agrees with the literature.[6] Assuming that the gender ratio in PWS is close to unity, as the two previous studies found, it therefore seemed that most of any missing cases (estimate 14 to 30) would be female. This is not surprising; at all ages, suspicion of PWS is more likely in males because of hypogonadism in childhood and short stature with obesity in adulthood. However, in two of the three age groups in which females did in fact out-number males, the age group was in the over 30s, raising the possibility that with PWS, as in the general population, women outlive men. Given the assumptions about those with PWS not identified, we suggested that a population prevalence of 1:52 000 is a lower bound and that the true prevalence is somewhat higher, nearer to 1:45 000.

Unlike the two previous population surveys of PWS, the present survey was large enough to allow the age structure of the PWS population to be examined. We were able to estimate both birth incidence and mortality rate. The estimate of mortality rate assumes that there is no systematic age-related ascertainment bias. For example, the age data might have been stepped corresponding to advances in awareness and diagnostic refinements, but the age structure found argued against such a cohort effect. However, it is possible that there were older adults with PWS born before the syndrome was well known and in which the diagnosis was never considered. Whilst this possibility cannot be ruled out, we argued that an increased mortality rate is the most likely explanation of the age profile of this

Table 4.4. Estimated birth
incidence, population
prevalence and mortality data

Birth incidence 1:20 000
Population prevalence 1:52 000
Mortality rate 3% per year

population-based cohort of people with PWS. High rates of both physical and psychiatric disorder have been reported,[7] and preliminary analysis of further data from this study provides evidence of significant morbidity. It seemed likely that obesity and associated complications were the main contributory factor. However, a systematic prospective study is required to establish whether this is the case or not. The physical health needs of people with learning disability are often not properly assessed or adequately met,[8] and disorders such as Type 2 diabetes mellitus might easily be missed in this population. There is also concern that misguided support strategies in adult life may result in marked weight increase and that resultant obesity-related problems then occur.[9,10]

Our birth incidence findings are in line with those from a recent report from Australia, which estimated birth incidence there to be 1:25 000 live births per year.[11] This was based on 30 live births of genetically confirmed PWS babies reported to the Australian Paediatric Surveillance Unit between 1998 and 2000. This is a lower bound, since some cases may have been missed or not reported, and it is based on only three years' data. The main findings reported in this chapter are summarised in Table 4.4.

REFERENCES

1. Butler, M. G. Prader–Willi syndrome: current understanding of cause and diagnosis. *American Journal of Medical Genetics* **35** (1990), 319–332.
2. Akefeldt, A., Gillberg, C. & Larsson, C. Prader–Willi syndrome in a Swedish rural county: epidemiological aspects. *Developmental Medicine and Child Neurology* **33** (1991), 715–721.
3. Burd, L., Vesely, B., Martsolf, J. & Kerbeshian, J. Prevalence study of Prader–Willi syndrome in North Dakota. *American Journal of Medical Genetics* **37** (1990), 97–99.
4. Glenn, C. C., Saitoh, S., Jong, M. T. C. *et al.* Gene structure, DNA methylation, and imprinted expression of the human *SNRPN* gene. *American Journal of Human Genetics* **58** (1996), 335–346.
5. Akefeldt, A., Anvret, M., Grandell, U., Norliner, R. & Gillberg, C. Parental exposure to hydrocarbons in Prader–Willi syndrome. *Developmental Medicine and Child Neurology* **37** (1995), 1101–1109.

6. Cassidy, S. B., Forsythe, M., Heeger, S. *et al.* comparison of phenotype between patients with Prader–Willi syndrome due to deletion 15q and uniparental disomy 5. *American Journal of Medical Genetics* **68** (1997), 433–440.

7. Greenswag, L. R. Adults with Prader–Willi syndrome: a survey of 232 cases. *Developmental Medicine and Child Neurology* **29** (1987), 145–152.

8. Lennox, N. G. & Kerr, M. P. Primary health care and people with an intellectual disability: the evidence base. *Journal of Intellectual Disability Research* **41** (2000), 365–372.

9. Dykens, E. M., Goff, B. J., Hodapp, R. M. *et al.* Eating themselves to death: have 'personal rights' gone too far in treating people with Prader–Willi syndrome? *Mental Retardation* **35** (1997), 312–314.

10. Holland, A. J. & Wong, J. Genetically-determined obesity in Prader–Willi syndrome: the ethics and legality of treatment. *Journal of Medical Ethics* **25** (1999), 230–236.

11. Smith, A., Egan, J., Ridley, G. *et al.* Birth prevalence of Prader–Willi syndrome in Australia. *Archives of Disease in Childhood* **88** (2003), 263–264.

5

Relationship between genetic and clinical diagnosis

In Chapter 1, we outlined the events leading up to the adoption of the Consensus Diagnostic Criteria (CDC).[1] A weighted score of eight or more for ages four years and above (five or more for ages less than four years), based on the presence of eight major (score 1) and 11 minor (score 0.5) symptoms, is considered sufficient for a clinical diagnosis of PWS. According to these diagnostic criteria, there is no requirement that any particular one (or more) of the criteria are present, rather that the total number present exceeds a given threshold. This was a relaxation of the implicit criteria of individual physicians. As noted in Chapter 1, some early reports, such as Hall & Smith[2] and Pipes & Holm,[3] did consider that the presence of some criteria were critical in the diagnosis of PWS.

Before PWS was recognised as a genetic syndrome, diagnosis was necessarily based on clinical criteria, and the primary role of such criteria was to ensure as accurate a diagnostic process as possible. When it was recognised that at least half of the people diagnosed with PWS had a deletion on the long arm of chromosome 15, clinical criteria and genetic criteria were used interchangeably. More recently, with the major advances made in the genetics of PWS, genetic testing for PWS has become the definitive diagnostic tool. The clinical diagnostic criteria are still of major importance, but their role has changed from firm diagnosis to that of raising a suspicion of PWS.[4] In the context of this new role, it is important to know which of the criteria are associated with the greatest probability of a genetic diagnosis of PWS. The association between genotype and phenotype is also important from a more theoretical perspective. As yet, the mechanisms that link genotype to phenotype are poorly understood and whether one or more genes are involved is yet unclear. Study of the relationship between the spectrum of major, minor and supportive diagnostic criteria and variations at the genotypic level would help clarify this. Fundamentally, the issue is whether all the manifestations of PWS can be explained by a single mechanism and, by implication, abnormal or absent expression of a single maternally imprinted gene, or whether very diverse mechanisms are involved, suggesting that PWS is truly a contiguous gene syndrome in which the absence of expression of more than one imprinted gene is required to give rise to the full phenotype.

Current understanding of genetics

It is clear from the literature that great strides have been made into the genetics of PWS in the last 20 years or so. An outline of some of the discoveries appears in Chapter 1. But there are still a great many outstanding questions. How many and which genes are involved? What are the associated gene products? How do these cause the characteristic features of the syndrome? Why is there variation of the phenotype in regard to these characteristic features within genetic subtypes? What do phenotypic differences between the subtypes tell us about the genetics of PWS or about particular genes on chromosome 15 (see Chapter 6)?

How many and which genes?

With regard to the first question, it is not known how many genes might be involved in PWS. The absence of expression of a single gene has been thought unlikely by geneticists to be the explanation, mainly because no person with PWS has been identified with a mutation of a single gene, other than those with mutations of the imprinting centre, the latter influencing the expression of more than one gene. A fault in the imprinting centre results in the paternal grandmother imprint failing to be reset, causing the imprinted genes on the paternal chromosome to carry a maternal imprint, thus imitating a disomy. However, the possibility of a mutation affecting a specific gene within the PWS critical region, the absence of expression of which leads to PWS, has not been ruled out.

Additional circumstantial evidence of multiple gene involvement is found in the wide range of characteristics in the PWS phenotype. However, it is of note that the complex phenotype of Angelman syndrome is due to the absence of expression of a single paternally imprinted gene on chromosome 15. Thus, the complexity of a phenotype may be due to post-transcriptional effects rather than the influence of the absence of expression of more than one gene.

Speculation continues on the possible identity of the PWS gene(s). Fewer than 10 paternally expressed genes have so far been identified in the PWS critical region, including *MAGEL2*, *NECDIN* (NDN), the zinc-finger protein (*ZNF127*), *IPW*, and the small ribonucleoprotein N (*SNRPN*) with its partner *SNURF* (or *SNRPN* upstream reading frame). There are also nine paternally expressed transcription units of unknown function. These include *ZNF127AS*, *PAR1*, *PAR5* and *PARSN*,[5] and the *SNRPN* gene also has several upstream exons that can be differentially spliced to produce imprinting centre specific transcripts. It has been estimated that the PWS region might contain as many as 100 imprinted or non-imprinted genes. The imprinting centre covers about 100 kb of genomic sequence but is bipartite in structure as deletions of the proximal portion result in Angelman syndrome, while deletion of the distal portion is associated with PWS. The PWS imprinting control element spans the promotor and exon 1 of the *SNRPN* gene. The shortest region of overlap observed in imprinting centre mutations has been established with a size of about 4.3 kb. Under normal circumstances the PWS element switches the grand-maternal imprint to a paternal epigenotype in the father.

Some recent work on the genetics of the PWS region, based on both mouse and human studies, has centred on small nucleolar RNAs (SnoRNAs). Such genes are located in the nucleoli of cells, which are the sites of ribosomal RNA transcription and methylation modification, in which the SnoRNAs are involved. Some SnoRNA genes are transcribed independently, others are located within introns of protein-coding genes, most of whose functions are linked to translation. These latter SnoRNAs are co-transcribed with their host pre-mRNAs, and released by processing from excised introns. They contain the characteristic box C (UGAUGA) and box D (CUGA) motifs. In 2000, it was reported that three human SnoRNAs, expressed in brain tissue, map to the PWS region, and that *HBII-52* and *HBII-85* were absent from the cortex of a patient with PWS and from a PWS mouse model, demonstrating paternal imprinting status.[6] These SnoRNAs are encoded within introns of the large *SNURF–SNRPN* transcription unit, which spans more than 460 kb and contains at least 148 exons, including the *IPW* exons.[7]

What are the associated gene products?

Until the genes responsible and the associated gene products are identified the mode of causation of individual characteristics is unlikely to be fully understood. However, it is clear that many of the characteristics, such as those associated with the reproductive system, appetite and obesity, and short stature, are mediated through the hypothalamus, as discussed in Chapter 2. Thus, it would be predicted that any PWS gene(s) would be expressed in some or all of the hypothalamic nuclei, either in development and/or throughout life, in those without PWS but not in those with the syndrome. Research on the pathways linking the genotype via the brain to physical and behavioural characteristics can be carried out at any point in this chain. Indeed, it is research into the links from brain chemistry to the physical and behavioural characteristics end of this chain that is necessary in order to enable the development of interventions to alleviate some of the more distressing characteristics of PWS.

Why is there variation of the phenotype within genetic subtypes?

The observation of phenotypic variation within a syndrome is important, as such variation may help elucidate the underlying mechanisms and, specifically, whether there is a direct or indirect relationship between genotype and phenotype. In PWS a number of possible explanations of observed variation have been excluded over the years. These include the following explanations. First, that there are different genes for each characteristic and that the phenotype maps onto the variable patterns of expression of these genes. This explanation became untenable when the genes involved in PWS were shown to be imprinted and all the maternally imprinted genes in the PWS region were unexpressed. Second, it was briefly reported that genetic mosaicism occurred in PWS but this was found to be an error in the genetic technique. Third, imperfect or 'leaky' imprinting of the PWS gene(s) has also been proposed, whereby there would be variable levels of activity of imprinted genes between individuals with the syndrome. However, there has been no clear evidence to support this theoretical possibility, but the principle is important as, if shown to be the case, it could lead to novel therapeutic strategies in the future. Finally, based on the analyses of the data collected from the Cambridge study, we have proposed the 'threshold shift model'.[8] This model recognises that in the normal population there is a wide variation in most characteristics, including those characteristics that are at one extreme in PWS. People in general have different heights, have different levels of interest in food, tolerate different levels of pain without discomfort, and so on, and the distribution of these attributes in the general population usually has a normal distribution. Variation in the levels of some of these characteristics is often typical of family members. This is equally true of people with PWS. The difference between people with and without PWS is that those in the former group tend to be shifted towards one end of the spectrum; that is, the threshold of normality of a characteristic appears to be shifted towards one extreme and therefore occurs more frequently in that population. Our model postulates that the effect of the PWS genotype is, at least for some of the characteristics, to bring about this threshold shift and that the apparent variation in prevalence of PWS characteristics is merely normal variation of a shifted threshold.[8] If this is correct, then it is important to identify those characteristics that are universal (e.g. eating disorder) and those that are highly prevalent, but not universal (e.g. skin-picking, obsessions). In the former there is likely to be a more direct relationship between abnormal gene expression and the characteristic, and in the latter the observed prevalence may reflect the above postulated mechanism.

Previous investigations of clinical versus genetic criteria

A key clinical issue is whether there are certain clinical diagnostic features, which if present or absent, predict with a high degree of certainty, a positive or negative genetic diagnosis. Previous reports describing the relationship between groups of diagnostic criteria and a positive genetic diagnosis of PWS have suggested that no such necessary criteria exist. Gillessen-Kaesbach et al.[9] compared the PWS genetic subtypes, deletions, and disomies on a number of diagnostic criteria and physical measurements in 167 people with PWS. They found only one characteristic that was always present in any group, namely, cryptorchidism in disomy males. However, it is not clear from the report how the presence or not of the clinical criteria were determined, since those with PWS ranged in age from 1 month to 33 years. Presumably at least some data came from parental reports, but under what circumstances? The same authors also describe a series of 450 genetics tests on people referred as possibly having PWS.[10] Of the 58 people examined personally, only 28 were considered to have PWS. Clinical data on the other 392 people genetically tested was gathered by questionnaire. Among the 28 people personally examined and genetically confirmed as having PWS, all were reported as being hypotonic at birth, having hypogenitalism and the characteristic facial appearance. All but one, aged 26 months, had reported feeding problems, all those over 26 months had hyperphagia, and all but one, aged 7 years, had global developmental delay and/or 'mental retardation'. Among those older than 26 months, only one, a child with isodisomy aged 6 years, had no behavioural problems. Buchholz et al.[11] described 115 people with suspected PWS referred for genetic testing. Clinical data was collected by personal observation supplemented by questionnaire, letter or telephone discussions. On the basis of this clinical data, the people with possible PWS were subdivided into four groups by clinical diagnostic scores: 26 people scored eight or over (classical phenotype); 15 scored between five and eight (possible); 62 people scored below five (unlikely); and the final 12 were described as hypotonic babies. All those given a diagnosis of PWS on genetic testing belonged to the classical phenotype or hypotonic babies groups. The prevalence of individual symptoms in each group was not given so it is not possible to say whether any particular symptom was always present. In the Livieri et al.[12] study, clinical criteria were collected by questionnaire on 82 people genetically diagnosed as having PWS. None of the criteria were universally present. The highest prevalence rates were 98% in the case of cryptorchidism and 92% for neonatal hypotonia.

Clinical diagnostic criteria in the Cambridge study

As described in Chapter 3, the Cambridge study tried to cover a large range of topics relevant to people with PWS and there had to be some compromise between the extent of data collection and the willingness of informants and people with PWS to be part of the study. For this reason it was decided to accept the judgement of informants, confirmed where possible by the researchers, as to the presence or not of the various criteria. So, for example, the criterion 'small hands or feet' was considered present if the informant (and researchers) judged that it was so, rather than taking actual measurements. The only measurement actually made that was relevant to the clinical criteria was the height of the person with PWS, which was required for the calculation of Body Mass Index. Two of the CDC criteria, specific facial characteristics and a straight ulnar border to the hands, were considered to be so subjective that they were not included in the Cambridge list. The appendix to this chapter compares the criteria of the CDC with those of the Cambridge study.

Early criteria for PWS were mainly physiological, but the CDC contains items relating to behaviour. Hyperphagia and skin picking are included as separate items, while another item specifies five or more of the following characteristic behaviour problems: temper tantrums; violent outbursts; obsessive–compulsive behaviour; tendency to be argumentative; oppositional; rigid; manipulative; possessive; stubborn; perseverating; stealing; and lying. Indeed, questionnaire-based studies have shown that people with PWS have a characteristic behavioural profile in which outbursts of temper (including aggressive behaviour and screaming), self harm (especially skin picking), mood swings and repetitive speech are common[13] (see Chapter 8). Repetitive questioning, compulsive behaviours and hoarding are also common, and it has been proposed that people with PWS are at increased risk for obsessive–compulsive disorder[14] (see Chapter 11). Adaptive behaviours, measured by the Vineland Adaptive Behaviour Scales,[15] show strengths in the Daily Living Skills domain and weaknesses in the Socialisation domain.[16] The most striking behaviour is that of severe and persistent over-eating which, if unrestricted, leads to life-threatening obesity.[17] These behaviours were itemised separately in the main questionnaire of the Cambridge study and in the Vineland scales (see Chapter 3).

The Cambridge investigation of clinical versus genetic criteria

We examined more closely the relationship between clinical and genetic diagnoses in a large number of people with established or suspected PWS. This chapter reports agreements and disagreements between clinical and genetic diagnoses. We consider whether a genetic diagnosis implies the presence of any one (or more) of the major, minor or supportive diagnostic criteria, and also whether the presence of any one (or more) particular diagnostic criteria implies a positive genetic finding, and what minimal genetic findings correspond to a positive finding on the basis of the clinical diagnostic criteria. In this chapter we also report on four specific cases that illustrate diagnostic difficulties in the absence of genetic testing. An early diagnosis of PWS is of particular importance as the propensity to over-eat can start as early as two years of age, and parental control of access to food can prevent the development of life-threatening obesity. In addition, we also found high rates of physical morbidity and mortality that are likely to be preventable if weight is adequately controlled[18,19] (see Chapter 9). Thus, an early suspicion of the diagnosis followed by genetic testing is important.

Unlike the previous studies, described above, the Cambridge study had the advantage of direct interviews rather than relying on questionnaire-based information. Also, the research team were deliberately over-inclusive in the initial selection of people who might possibly have PWS, and recruited a significant number of people with obesity syndromes who were subsequently found to be genetically negative for PWS. Thus, the specificity of particular diagnostic symptoms to PWS, compared to those with other causes for their obesity, can be considered. In addition, a comparison group of people with learning disabilities not due to PWS has been included, and therefore symptoms that might be considered potentially diagnostic of PWS, but are in fact associated with having a learning disability in general and are not specific to PWS, can be identified.

The study cohorts

The people involved in this particular investigation came from three sources: the original population nominees; volunteers who had or might have PWS recruited from outside the population region; and people with learning disabilities but not PWS, who were recruited as a comparison group. The people from these three sources were divided into three groups: those with genetically confirmed PWS (PWS group); those who were genetically negative but fulfilled clinical criteria for PWS or where some clinical data were missing (e.g. parents were dead or could not remember or the person was adopted) but they had previously been given a 'PWS' label (PWS-like group); and those who met neither the genetic nor the clinical criteria or were recruited as comparisons and were presumed not to meet genetic criteria (comparison group). Of the original 93 people who agreed to take part in the phenotypic study, 61 were confirmed as meeting genetic criteria for PWS (see Genetic diagnosis section below) and 19 had negative genetic findings. The remaining 13 did not give blood samples and had no previous positive genetic records. Six of the negative genetic participants also failed to meet clinical criteria, as did four of the 13 who did not give blood samples (criteria score <5). These people were included in the comparison group. Thirteen of the people who had negative genetic findings and nine who did not give blood samples either met clinical criteria or where some clinical data were missing (e.g. parents were dead or could not remember or the person was adopted) but they had previously been given a 'PWS' label. The former 13 people were put in the PWS-like group and the nine who did not give blood samples were omitted. Additional people said to have PWS were recruited from outside the region in an effort to increase the numbers in the study with the rarer genetic subtypes of PWS. Of these, 42 had positive genetic tests (PWS group) and six had negative genetics but clinical criteria were positive (criteria score >5), or missing (PWS-like group). In addition, a comparison group of 22 people with learning disabilities of other (mixed) aetiologies (no blood samples requested) was recruited to augment the 10 people from the original 93 who clearly met neither clinical nor genetic criteria. The derivation of the various samples is shown in Figure 5.1.

Measures used

As described in Chapter 3, the semi-structured interview included questions about the presence or absence of most of the diagnostic criteria (see Appendix 3.1), and supplementary questions were used to clarify answers or to seek examples (e.g. shoe size, examples of high pain threshold). As these data were largely gathered retrospectively from parents (and in many cases they were making judgements with respect to siblings), we divided positive endorsements into 'very positive' and 'positive'. This may have created a false division, depending on parental style and memory, as we noted in Chapter 3. Similarly, the definitions of the different severity of reported behaviours were operationalised and divided into those considered 'very bad' (on the basis of frequency and/or severity), 'bad' (worse than normal), or 'absent' (no worse than normal). The assessments of cognitive function and attainments provided verification of learning disabilities in all participants.

The same assessments and interviews, by the same two researchers, were used for all groups, thus removing some possible sources of variation in the data.

Genetic diagnosis

Blood samples were later obtained, or genetic records accessed, from all people suspected of having PWS who gave their consent (i.e. interviews were conducted blind to genetic findings). The blood samples were sent to the same geneticist. Methylation analysis was undertaken at the *SNURF–SNRPN* locus and a genetic diagnosis of PWS confirmed if only a maternal band was detected.[20] Cytogenetic analysis was then used to establish whether a deletion was present and parental samples were

GROUP 1: PWS genetics positive

> 61 population sample (49 blood samples received, 12 genetic records)
> 42 from other areas (33 blood samples received, 9 genetic records)

GROUP 2: PWS genetics negative; clinical criteria positive or missing

> 13 population sample (13 blood samples received)
>
> 6 from other areas (6 blood samples received)

GROUP 3: Clinical criteria negative

> 10 population sample (6 blood samples received)
>
> 22 learning disabled controls

OMITTED: Clinical criteria positive or missing; no blood tests

> 9 population sample

Figure 5.1.   Characteristics of contrast groups.

requested to confirm disomies. Microsatellite analysis at 10 or more loci spanning the entire deletion region from D15S11 to D15S219 was also undertaken for all samples. In contrast, the genetics records accessed often contained only a positive genetic diagnosis on the basis of methylation pattern and no information on genetic subtype.

Analyses undertaken

Frequencies of clinical diagnostic symptoms and characteristic PWS behaviours were obtained for the three groups: PWS; PWS-like; and comparison group. Nine people are missing from this analysis as no blood samples were obtained and no genetic records were available. In the first group, prevalences of the various characteristics were compared for the population sample only and then the full sample. Discriminant analyses were performed for the following contrast groups: PWS v. Comparison; and PWS v. Combined PWS-like and Comparison. Phenotypic and behavioural differences between deletion and disomy forms of PWS are reported elsewhere (see Chapters 6 and 7).

Case studies

To illustrate some of the problems involved in linking genetic and clinical findings four people are described whose symptomatology or genetics are similar to PWS but in other ways are atypical. These include: (1) a 32-year-old man with negative genetics but a very positive clinical diagnosis; (2) a 22-year-old man with normal *SNRPN* methylation but with a small deletion in the PWS region (del 15q12); (3) a 36-year-old man with normal chromosome 15 findings but with a deletion on chromosome 6 (del 6); and (4) a 18-year-old woman with positive PWS genetics and with our 'core' clinical features but with very few behavioural symptoms and an IQ of 103.

Results

In the genetically positive group, and in the PWS-like group identified above, we found two pervasive characteristics. First, there was the eating disturbance associated with the syndrome. Although some mothers denied having problems with their son's or daughter's eating behaviours, when questioned further, all admitted that their offspring could not cope with total independence. Where people with PWS and apparent self-control over their eating behaviour had tried to live independently, weight had always become a severe problem. Second, even when IQ was above 70 (19.6% of our population sample), there were impairments in social cognition, flexibility, comprehension of abstract ideas and concepts of time and number.

In Table 5.1 the prevalence rates of individual clinical diagnostic criteria (including specific behaviours) are given for the PWS, PWS-like, and comparison groups. We note that the population sample of people with PWS is included in the full PWS sample, which did not differ statistically from the population sample in the prevalence of any criterion (data not shown). Indeed, differences in criterion prevalence rates between the population and full samples were zero for the 'core' criteria, which had prevalence rates of 100%. Learning disabilities are not included, since these were common to all groups. We also note that some

Table 5.1. Endorsement of clinical criteria in genetic subgroups

Criterion	Genetics positive ($n = 103$) all clinically positive			Genetics negative, ($n = 19$) clinical criteria +ve/missing			Genetics negative, ($n = 32$) clinical criteria negative		
	Yes	Mild	No	Yes	Mild	No	Yes	Mild	No
Severe floppiness	96	5	0	10	1	2	4	4	22
Poor suck	94	5	0	7	1	5	4	1	25
Difficulty feeding	98	2	0	11	1	3	11	1	19
Decreased movement	65	7	23	6	1	4	2	3	20
Weak cry/Inactive	94	6	0	7	4	2	2	4	22
Childhood obesity	77	4	18	13	2	2	17	2	12
Overeat/food obsession	78	12	11	15	3	0	18	3	10
Hypogonadism	54	0	0	5	0	1	4	1	9
Periods per year	22	8	0	1	0	6	1	0	7
Disturbed/Noisy sleep	56	10	34	14	2	3	13	2	16
Short height	73	1	23	14	0	3	10	0	21
Fair for family	7	49	43	1	7	7	2	11	18
Small hands or feet	85	11	3	8	3	5	6	7	16
Eye problems	74	1	24	14	0	3	17	0	14
Thick saliva	55	23	21	3	2	14	1	3	27
Articulation problems	65	16	16	9	4	2	17	4	10
High pain threshold	50	29	10	6	7	2	3	13	11
Temperature insensitive	44	11	30	8	1	7	3	1	22
Skill with jigsaws	28	14	48	0	3	15	0	3	28
Stubborn	80	14	3	16	3	0	18	5	9
Scoliosis	30	8	62	2	1	16	0	4	28
Reduced vomiting	46	39	10	0	7	10	4	7	19
Severity eating	45	24	27	4	8	5	3	10	18
Possessive	47	31	24	7	5	7	11	8	12
Skin picking	56	19	25	8	5	5	3	9	20
Temper tantrums	63	26	4	11	2	2	15	9	8
Repeated questions	63	12	20	12	3	2	7	5	18
Obsessional behaviour	66	26	6	10	7	0	8	14	10
Violent behaviour	34	33	28	9	2	6	11	6	15
Mood swings	34	18	48	8	5	5	6	7	19
Argumentative	37	28	27	8	0	6	12	5	13
Lying	34	25	32	3	6	5	9	7	12
Stealing	40	23	30	8	7	3	6	4	21

clinical features and behaviours are almost as common in the learning disabilities group, and especially in the PWS-like group, as in the PWS group and should probably not be considered as characteristic of PWS so much as of learning disability.

Some clinical features appeared always to be present (floppy at birth, weak cry or inactivity, poor suck, feeding difficulties, hypogonadism – see Appendix 5.1) whenever genetic testing indicated abnormal methylation at *SNRPN*. A definite 'no' to the question of whether any of these features were present was sufficient to ensure the finding of a normal methylation pattern (i.e. negative genetics for PWS). On the other hand, seven out of 51 (six of 19 in Group 2 and one of 32 in Group 3) of people with normal methylation fulfilled the first four of these criteria and three males and one adult female also had hypogonadism. This is quite a high rate of 'false positives' if we use these criteria alone, and we investigated whether a different subset of criteria might discriminate better than this.

Table 5.2 shows the result of the discriminant analyses between (a) the PWS group and the comparison group and (b) the PWS group and the combined PWS-like and comparison groups. There was too much missing data in the PWS-like group to do a three-way discriminant analysis. The first of these analyses, between genetically confirmed PWS and people with learning disabilities of other aetiology and without clinical suspicion of PWS, shows that 99% of people with PWS were correctly classified using four criteria: *floppy at birth; weak cry/inactivity of infant; poor suck at birth;* and *childhood obesity*. The second analysis shows that four variables: *poor suck at birth; weak cry/inactivity of infant; decreased vomiting;* and *thick saliva,* best discriminated between genetically confirmed PWS and all other learning disabled, but correct classification fell to 92% of cases.

We also considered the issue of clinical diagnosis in later life when clinical information from birth may not be available (ie. the first five items of the Appendix 5.1). Table 5.3 shows the results of four discriminant analyses: (A) and (B) between the PWS group and the comparison group and (C) and (D) between the PWS group and the combined PWS-like and comparison groups. Infancy data is omitted from all four discriminants and also hypogonadism from (A) and (C). The first two of these analyses, between genetically confirmed PWS and learning disabilities of other aetiology and without clinical suspicion of PWS, shows that 94% of cases were correctly classified using two criteria, *small hands or feet* and *hypogonadism* in (A) and four criteria, *small hands or feet, thick saliva, not feeling hot/cold, stubborn > usual* in (B). The other analyses show that the latter four variables best discriminated in (C) and *hypogonadism, small hands or feet,* and *thick saliva* best discriminated in (D) between genetically confirmed PWS and all other learning disabled, but correct classification fell to 86–92% of cases.

Table 5.2. Variables which best discriminate between positive and negative genetic diagnoses of Prader–Willi syndrome

(A) PWS +ve Genet v. Control

50 PWS +ve, and 15 control had full data

Classification results

Action Step Entered	No. of variables in	Wilks' Lambda	Sig.	Actual group	No. of cases	Predicted group 1	2
1 Floppy at birth	1	0.14863	0.0000	Group 1	95	95	0
2 Weak cry/inactive	2	0.09996	0.0000			100%	0%
3 Poor suck at birth	3	0.08388	0.0000	Group 2	26	1	25
4 Childhood obesity	4	0.07439	0.0000			3.8%	96.2%
				Ungrouped	19	14	5
						73.7%	26.3%
-				Percent of 'grouped' cases correctly classified: 99.2%			

(B) PWS +ve Genet v. PWS −ve

Genet combined with Control

50 PWS +ve, 4 PWS −ve and 15 control had full data

control had full data

Classification results

Action Step Entered	No. of variables in	Wilks' Lambda	Sig.	Actual group	No. of cases	Predicted group 1	2
1 Poor suck at birth	1	0.28916	0.0000	Group 1	89	87	2
2 Weak cry/inactive	2	0.17886	0.0000			97.8%	2.2%
3 Vomiting	3	0.16721	0.0000	Group 2	38	8	30
4 Thick saliva	4	0.15756	0.0000			21.1%	78.90%
				Ungrouped	7	6	1
						85.7%	14.3%
				Percent of 'grouped' cases correctly classified: 92.1%			

As an indication of the possible relationships between clinical criteria and genetics, four unusual cases are presented, all of which come from our population sample. Case (2) is certainly more positive on the diagnostic criteria than cases (1) and (4); case (3) is positive on the diagnostic criteria, but lacks one of the 'core' characteristics. Table 5.4 shows the prevalence of clinical diagnostic criteria (including behaviours) in the four cases:

1. Normal methylation and expression at *SNRPN* but deleted at 15q12 (probe p1R39) in the PWS region (included as PWS since there is a deletion in the PWS region, as noted in a previous genetic record and confirmed as part of this study).

Table 5.3. Variables excluding infancy data which best discriminate between positive and negative genetic diagnoses of Prader–Willi syndrome

(A) PWS +ve Genet v. Control Hypogonadism excluded

53 PWS +ve, and 16 control had full data

Classification results

Action Step Entered	No. variables in	Wilks' Lambda	Sig.	Actual group	No. of cases	Predicted group 1	2
1 Small hands or feet	1	0.47241	0.0000	Group 1	78	73	5
2 Thick saliva	2	0.34721	0.0000			93.6%	6.4%
3 Not feel hot/cold	3	0.29825	0.0000	Group 2	22	1	21
4 Stubborn > usual	4	0.27820	0.0000			4.5%	95.5%
				Ungrouped	18	12	6
						66.7%	33.3%
-				Percent of 'grouped' cases correctly classified: 94.0%			

(B) PWS +ve Genet v. Control Hypogonadism included

42 PWS +ve and 12 control had full data

Classification results

Action Step Entered	No. variables in	Wilks' Lambda	Sig.	Actual group	No. of cases	Predicted group 1	2
1 Hypogonadism	1	0.22736	0.0000	Group 1	80	79	1
2 Small hands or feet	2	0.15904	0.0000			98.8%	1.3%
				Group 2	22	5	17
						22.7%	77.3%
				Ungrouped	20	13	7
						65%	35%
				Percent of 'grouped' cases correctly classified: 94.1%			

(C) PWS +ve Genet v. PWS −ve Genet combined with Control Hypogonadism excluded

53 PWS +ve, 4 PWS −ve and 16 control had full data

Classification results

Action Step Entered	No. variables in	Wilks' Lambda	Sig.	Actual group	No. of cases	Predicted group 1	2
1 Small hands or feet	1	0.48512	0.0000	Group 1	88	82	6
2 Thick saliva	2	0.35625	0.0000			93.2%	6.8%
3 Vomiting	3	0.31691	0.0000	Group 2	41	12	29
4 Stubborn > usual	4	0.29990	0.0000			29.3%	70.7%
				Ungrouped	8	5	3
						62.5%	37.5%
				Percent of 'grouped' cases correctly classified: 86.1%			

Table 5.3. (*cont.*)

(D) PWS +ve Genet v. PWS −ve Genet combined with Control Hypogonadism included

42 PWS +ve, 3 PWS −ve and 12 control had full data

Classification results

Action Step Entered	No. variables in	Wilks' Lambda	Sig.	Actual group	No. of cases	Predicted group 1	2
1 Hypogonadism	1	0.44567	0.0000	Group 1	77	76	1
2 Small hands or feet	2	0.29624	0.0000			98.7%	1.3%
3 Thick saliva	3	0.27508	0.0000	Group 2	33	8	25
						24.2%	75.8%

Percent of 'grouped' cases correctly classified: 91.8%

2. Genetically normal at the PWS region (see Genetic diagnosis) but clinically very positive.
3. Genetically normal chromosome 15 but deletion on chromosome 6.
4. Abnormal methylation and expression at *SNRPN*, but has no behavioural problems and an IQ of 103.

The initial suspicion that an infant or child might have PWS is raised because of the presence or not of particular clinical characteristics. As we noted earlier, the purpose of clinical diagnostic criteria has shifted from making the diagnosis to raising the suspicion of PWS. Our aim here is to try to refine the use of the criteria in this respect. Our results show that, in both our population sample and in our augmented sample of people with PWS, there appear to be core symptoms that are always present in the case of a positive genetic diagnosis. In our findings, a definite 'no' to any one of these criteria implies a normal methylation pattern. However, the data in Table 5.1, the discriminant analysis, and case (2) all show that they are not sufficient, in that their presence does not predict with certainty the genetic diagnosis of PWS. Moreover, we were unable to find a set of clinical criteria that were sufficient to predict a positive genetic finding, although the predictive power of the above four 'core' criteria was greater than 90%.

The methodology used in our study may account for the differences between our results and those in previous published studies (in which our 'core' criteria, although most strongly endorsed, were not always present in 100% of cases). Not only did we use semi-structured interviews, conducted in an informal manner in the clients' own homes, but the same two people carried out all the interviews. If we had not used our interview method, but had used Yes/No questionnaires, we believe that our results would have been less clear. For example, three mothers said that their babies were 'stiff' at birth but became 'very floppy' within hours and had to be tube fed. Ideally, we would have liked hospital records of the babies' conditions

Table 5.4. Four case studies

	Case 1	Case 2	Case 3	Case 4
Major criteria				
Severe floppiness at birth with later improvement	Yes Some	Yes	Yes	Yes
Poor suck at birth with later improvement	Yes Some	Yes	Yes	Yes
Difficulty feeding at birth	Yes	Yes	Yes	Yes
Obesity during childhood -(age when noticed)	Yes(2)	Yes(3)	Yes(1.25)	Yes(8)
Hypogonadism-with any of the following, depending on age:	Yes	Yes	No	Yes
Males: undescended testes, surgery on testes, decreased facial and body hair, lack of voice change/age at voice change, early pubertal signs	No Yes	Yes Yes	No No	
Females: does/did she have periods (no if only when on pill), age of first period, how many periods per year, early pubertal signs				No
Learning difficulties	Yes	Yes	Yes	No MR
Tendency to overeat/obsession with food (from age)	Yes(2.5)	Yes(2)	Yes(2)	No
Deletion 15q11–13 on high resolution (>650 bands) or other cytogenetic/ molecular abnormality of the PWS chromosome region, including maternal disomy	Yes del 15q12 Meth.normal	No Meth.normal	No del on 6 Meth.normal	Yes Small del Meth.PWS
Minor criteria				
Decreased movement of baby during pregnancy	Yes	Yes	Yes	Yes
Weak cry or inactivity as a baby	Yes	Yes	Some	Yes
Frequency and severity of any: temper tantrums, repetitive questioning, obsessional behaviour, violent/aggressive behaviour, fluctuations in mood, argumentative, lying, stealing, stubborn, any other behaviour problems	6	9	8	2
Disturbed or noisy sleep	Yes	Yes	Yes	No
Short height:	No?	Yes	No	Yes
Growth hormone ever	No	Yes	No	Yes

Table 5.4. (*cont.*)

	Case 1	Case 2	Case 3	Case 4
Hypopigmentation-fair skin and hair compared to family	Sandy hair	Fair skin	No	No
Small hands or feet	Yes	Yes	Hands	Hands
Eye problems (short sight, long sight, squint)	Yes	Yes	Yes	No
Thick saliva with crusting at corners of mouth	No	No	No	No
Difficulty with articulating words	Yes	Yes	Yes	Yes
Skin picking	Yes	Yes	Yes	Some
Supportive findings				
High pain threshold	Yes	Yes	Yes	Some
Decreased vomiting; Ever vomited: frequency	Little	Little	Little	Never
Not feeling hot or cold: abnormal temperature response	Yes	Yes	?	?
Scoliosis or spinal curvature	No	No	No	No
Unusual skill with jigsaw puzzles	Yes	No	No	Yes

at birth, but this was not possible in the present study. Although anecdotal we were impressed by the number of first-time mothers who said they had known that 'something was wrong' during pregnancy (less surprisingly, most of those mothers with experience of previous pregnancies reported similar feelings).

A second advantage of this study is that it was based on a population sample and the prevalences of the various clinical criteria in the full sample could be compared with those of the population. (All of the 'core' criteria were present in 100% in both, and the prevalence of other criteria were very similar in the population and the full sample of PWS.) This report is therefore more likely than most reports in the literature to be representative of PWS.

Genetic tests for PWS have not always been made, especially in the past, when symptoms have been suggestive. This may have been due to a number of factors including ignorance of the syndrome, the cost of genetic analyses and the possible unnecessary emotional upset to the parents if the suspicion were not confirmed. Clearly, we need to include all positive cases and as few negative cases as possible in the set of people tested for PWS. All positive cases are included in the set of people with all of the 'core' symptoms. Our investigations indicate two circumstances, for infants and for older people respectively, in which genetic tests for PWS should be made. All of the 'core criteria' identified above can be recognised in the first few weeks of life in the case of males and all but one in the case of females. Therefore, if none of these criteria is definitely absent, a genetic test for PWS is clearly indicated. We estimated the cost of such a policy in terms of the number of negative genetic tests that might be involved. It would have resulted in one out of those 32 (3%) of our comparison group with learning disabilities with scores on all of these criteria being tested, and four out of 19 (21%) of those with PWS features but negative genetics. One fewer of these core criteria (four for males, three for females) would have added four more negative cases (6% and 11% respectively); two fewer would have added eight more cases (16% and 16% respectively). We also investigated indications for genetic testing later in life if data from the first weeks of life are missing. In these cases, indicators of PWS would be an eating disturbance and learning disabilities, as discussed above, with the following additional criterion. In the case of females, absent or infrequent (fewer than five per year) and sparse menses would appear to be a necessary symptom, and in the case of males undescended testes (in the absence of surgery) or small penis. Using this criterion, no positive genetic cases would have been missed, but two out of 15 females with negative genetics would have been included and 12 out of 25 males. Such cases should be increasingly rare, given the increasingly early age of diagnosis. Discriminant analysis (Table 5.3) showed that again no subset of criteria was sufficient to discriminate genetic cases. However, the results of the discriminant analyses indicated that certain criteria should be given more weight in diagnosis, either as core characteristics of PWS or as discriminators between PWS and other learning disabled groups.

Our findings also raise questions about more theoretical issues. Why do the core criteria have such high prevalences in all studies that look at genetically diagnosed PWS, and why is there such a variation in the prevalences within PWS of other criteria that distinguish PWS from other groups? The genetic test for PWS assumes that the genetic mechanisms identified to date are the only such mechanisms and operate through their effect on several specific imprinted genes. It is possible that the core clinical features of PWS are due to the failure of expression of a single gene and that a mutation in that gene would lead to the core clinical features of the syndrome. Thus, we cannot exclude the possibility that those with the core clinical features of PWS but apparently normal genetics for the PWS critical region, in fact have a mutation in the putative 'core' gene. This could also in principle be true for case 3, in which case the findings on chromosome 6 are an additional genetic abnormality. We believe this to be unlikely and, rather, that abnormalities at different genetic loci (as in Case 3) can give a similar clinical picture to that of PWS, as is clear from the literature.

The variable strengths of various PWS characteristics and behaviours have been explained elsewhere by our research group[8] in terms of natural genetic variation (usually resulting in a normal distribution of values in the population as a whole) combined with mechanisms we have described as 'all or none' (found in all people with PWS), 'threshold shift' (i.e. a distribution shifted in one direction relative to the general population so that only one tail conforms to acceptable values) and 'arrested development' (i.e. behaviour common to a certain developmental age that persists into adulthood in people with PWS) (see Chapter 8). The five core symptoms, together with an eating disturbance and learning disabilities, would then constitute the 'all or none' characteristics of PWS. Prevalence of characteristics such as 'a high pain threshold' and 'daytime sleepiness' would be explained by the threshold shift model, and typical PWS obsessive–compulsive behaviour (which is similar to that of normal children) would be explained by arrested development. The prevalence of a symptom explained by the 'threshold shift' model would then depend on the strength of that symptom relative to the normal population, and would be expected to vary between families as well as between individuals. It would be appropriate in scoring such a symptom to take account of family background.

Appendix 5.1

Comparison of Consensus Diagnostic Criteria with criteria ascertained in the Cambridge study

Consensus Diagnostic Criteria	Cambridge study Questionnaire
Major criteria	
Neonatal and infantile central hypotonia with poor suck, gradually improving with age	Severe floppiness at birth with later improvement
Feeding problems in infancy with need for special feeding techniques and poor weight gain/failure to thrive	Poor suck at birth with later improvement
	Difficulty feeding at birth (need for special feeding techniques)
Excessive or rapid weight gain on weight-for-length chart (excessive defined as crossing two centile channels) after 12 months but before 6 years of age; central obesity in the absence of intervention	Obesity during childhood – age when noticed, maximum weight ever and age when reached
Characteristic facial features with dolichocephaly in infancy, narrow face or bifrontal diameter, almond shaped eyes, small-appearing mouth with thin upper lip, down turned corners of the mouth (3 or more required)	
Hypogonadism-with any of the following, depending on age:	Males: undescended testes, surgery on testes, decreased facial and body hair, lack of voice change/age at voice change, early pubertal signs, small penis
(a) Genital hypoplasia male: scrotal hypoplasia, cryptorchidism, small penis and/or testes for age (<5th percentile) female: absence or severe hypoplasia of labia minora and/or clitoris	Females: does/did she have periods (no if only when on pill), age of first period, how many periods per year, early pubertal signs

(cont.)

(*cont.*)

Consensus Diagnostic Criteria	Cambridge study Questionnaire
(b) Delayed or incomlete gonadal maturation with delayed pubertal signs in the absence of intervention after 16yrs of age (male: small gonads, decreased facial and body hair lack of voice change; female: amenorrhea/oligomenorrhea after age 16)	
Global developmental delay in a child younger than 6 years of age; mild to moderate mental retardation or learning problems in older children	Learning difficulties
Hyperphagia/food foraging/obsession with food	Tendency to overeat/obsession with food
Deletion 15q11–13 on high resolution (>650 bands) or other cytogenetic/molecular abnormality of the PWS chromosome region, including maternal disomy	Genetic testing done, result of testing, where testing was done
Minor criteria	
Decreased fetal movement or infantile lethergy or weak cry in infancy, improving with age	Decreased movement of baby during pregnancy
	Weak cry or inactivity as a baby
Characteristic behaviour problems – temper tantrums, violent outbursts and obsessive-compulsive behaviour, tendency to be argumentative, oppositional, rigid, manipulative, possessive, and stubborn; perseverating, stealing, and lying (5 or more of these symptoms required)	Frequency and severity of any: temper tantrums, skin picking, repetitive questioning, obsessional behaviour, violent/aggressive behaviour, fluctuations in mood, argumentative, lying, stealing, stubborn, any other behaviour problems
Sleep disturbance or sleep apnoea	Disturbed or noisy sleep
Short stature for genetic background by age 15 (in the absence of growth hormone intervention)	Short height: heights of proband, mother, father, height centile. Growth hormone ever (dates)
Hypopigmentation-fair skin and hair compared to family	Fair skin and hair compared with family
Small hands (<25th centile) and/or feet (<10th centile) for height age	Small hands or feet (parents & researchers agree)
Narrow hands with straight ulnar border	
Eye abnormalities (esotropia, myopia)	Eye problems (short sight, long sight, squint)
Thick viscous saliva with crusting at corners of the mouth	Thick saliva with crusting at corners of mouth
Speech articulation defects	Difficulty with articulating words
Skin picking	
Supportive findings	
High pain threshold	High pain threshold (examples)
Decreased vomiting	Ever vomited: circumstances, frequency (0,<normal, normal)

(cont.)

Consensus Diagnostic Criteria	Cambridge study Questionnaire
Temperature instability in infancy or altered temperature sensitivity in older children and adults	Not feeling hot or cold when others are: abnormal temperature response
Scoliosis and/or kyphosis	Scoliosis or spinal curvature
Early adrenarche	
Osteoporosis	Thin bones e.g. easily broken
Unusual skill with jigsaw puzzles	Unusual skill with jigsaw puzzles
Normal neuromuscular studies	

REFERENCES

1. Holm, V. A., Cassidy, S. B., Butler, M. G. *et al.* Prader–Willi syndrome: consensus diagnostic criteria. *Pediatrics* **91** (1993), 398–402.
2. Hall, B. D. & Smith, D. W. Prader–Willi syndrome. A resume of 32 cases including an instance of affected first cousins, one of whom is of normal stature and intelligence. *Pediatrics* **81** (1972), 286–293.
3. Pipes, P. L. & Holm, V. A. Weight control of children with Prader–Willi syndrome. *Journal of the American Dietetic Association* **62** (1973), 520–524.
4. Gunay-Aygun, M., Schwartz, S., Heeger, S., O'Riordan, M. A. & Cassidy, S. B. The changing purpose of Prader–Willi syndrome clinical diagnostic criteria and proposed revised criteria. *Pediatrics* **108** (2001), e92.
5. Lee, S., Kozlov, S., Hernandez, L. *et al.* Expression and imprinting of *MAGEL2* suggest a role in Prader–Willi syndrome and the homologous murine imprinting phenotype. *Human Molecular Genetics* **9** (2000), 1813–1819.
6. Cavaille, J., Buiting, K., Kiefmann, M. *et al.* Identification of brain-specific and imprinted small nucleolar RNA genes exhibiting an unusual genomic organization. *Proceedings of the National Academy of Science of the USA* **97** (2000), 14311–14316.
7. Runte, M., Huttenhofer, A., Gross, S., Kiefmann, M., Horsthemke, B. & Buiting, K. The IC-SNURF-SNRPN transcript serves as a host for multiple small nucleolar RNA species and as an antisense RNA for UBE3A. *Human Molecular Genetics* **10** (2001), 2687–2700.
8. Holland, A. J., Whittington, J. E., Butler, J., Webb, T., Boer, H. & Clarke, D. Behavioural phenotypes associated with specific genetic disorders: evidence from a population-based study of people with Prader–Willi syndrome. *Psychological Medicine* **33** (2003), 141–153.
9. Gillessen-Kaesbach, G., Robinson, W., Lohmann, D., Kaya-Westerloh, S., Passarge, E. & Horsthemke, B. Genotype–phenotype correlation in a series of 167 deletion and non-deletion patients with Prader–Willi syndrome. *Human Genetics* **96** (1995), 638–643.
10. Gillessen-Kaesbach, G., Gross, S., Kaya-Westerloh, S., Passarge, E. & Horsthemke, B. DNA methylation based testing of 450 patients suspected of having Prader–Willi syndrome. *Journal of Medical Genetics* **32** (1995), 88–92.

11. Buchholz, T., Jackson, J., Robson, L. & Smith, A. Evaluation of methylation analysis for diagnostic testing in 258 referrals suspected of Prader–Willi or Angelman syndromes. *Human Genetics* **103** (1998), 535–539.

12. Livieri, C., Migliavacca, D., Piasenti C. *et al. Prevalence of minor criteria and supportive findings in patients with Prader–Willi syndrome.* Paper presented by the Genetic Obesity Study Group of the Italian Society of Pediatric Endocrinology and Diabetology at the 3rd triennial IPWSO scientific conference 1998, Venice, Italy.

13. Clarke, D. J., Boer, H., Chung, M. C. *et al.* Maladaptive behaviour in Prader–Willi syndrome in adult life. *Journal of Intellectual Disability Research* **40** (1996), 159–165.

14. Dykens, E. M., Hodapp, R. M., Walsh, K. & Nash, L. J. Adaptive and maladaptive behavior in Prader–Willi syndrome. *Journal of the American Academy of Child and Adolescent Psychiatry* **31** (1992), 1131–1135.

15. Sparrow, S. S., Balla, D. A. & Cicchetti, D. V. *Vineland Adaptive Behavior Scales.* Windsor. NFER-Nelson, 1984.

16. Dykens, E. M., Leckman, J. F. & Cassidy, S. B. Obsessions and compulsions in Prader–Willi syndrome. *Journal of Child Psychology and Psychiatry* **37** (1996), 995–1002.

17. Holland, A. J., Treasure, J., Coskeran, P., Dallow, J., Milton, N. & Hillhouse, E. Measurement of excessive appetite and metabolic changes in Prader–Willi syndrome. *International Journal of Obesity* **17** (1993), 526–532.

18. Whittington, J. E., Holland, A. J., Webb, T., Butler, J. V., Clarke, D. J. & Boer, H. Population prevalence and estimated birth incidence and mortality rate for people with Prader–Willi syndrome in one UK health region. *Journal of Medical Genetics* **38** (2001), 792–798.

19. Butler, J. V., Whittington, J. E., Holland, A. J., Webb, T., Clarke, D. J. & Boer, H. Prevalence of, and risk factors for, physical ill-health in people with Prader–Willi syndrome: a population-based study. *Developmental Medicine and Child Neurology* **44** (2002), 248–255.

20. American Society of Human Genetics/American College of Medical Genetics Test and Technology Transfer Committee. Diagnostic testing for Prader–Willi and Angelman syndromes: report of the ASHG/ACMG Test and Technology Transfer Committee. *American Journal of Human Genetics* **58** (1996), 1085–1088.

6

Phenotypic differences between the genetic subtypes

The two main genetic abnormalities that result in PWS are a chromosome 15q11–q13 deletion on the chromosome 15 of paternal origin and a chromosome 15 maternal disomy (see Chapter 1). The two other much rarer subtypes are a chromosomal re-arrangement (e.g. a translocation between chromosomes involving a break at 15q11–q13), and an imprinting centre defect on chromosome 15 (e.g. mutation or sub-microscopic deletion) that results in the equivalent of a disomy, in that both alleles of the imprinted genes have the same imprint (maternal in the case of PWS). In all four, the phenomenon of gender specific genomic imprinting is crucially important. PWS is among one of the best examples in humans where the expression of an allele of a gene depends upon whether it is inherited from the mother or father. In PWS, it is established that the gene or genes, whose absence of expression results in the syndrome, are only fully expressed when inherited from the father, but are quite normally imprinted (switched off) when inherited from the mother. It is proposed that genomic imprinting arose as a result of differential maternal/paternal evolutionary pressures.[1,2] In the case of such genes, in order for normal development to occur, the non-imprinted gene has to be present and transcriptionally active since the imprinted allele from the other parent, although present, is silenced and non-functional.[3] In the genetic subtypes of PWS the final common effect is that, for different genetic reasons, the normally active allele(s) of the putative PWS gene(s) are not expressed, either because they are absent (deleted) or because both alleles have the maternal imprint (i.e. are switched off) (see Figure 1.1).

Whilst all four genetic subtypes of PWS have a similar genetic effect, as described above, there are genotypic differences between them that may have phenotypic effects. Thus, comparison of the phenotypes of the genetic subtypes may be indicative of such genotype differences. For example, in those people with PWS due to a deletion, all of the non-imprinted genes also located within the deleted region are only present as a single copy. This is referred to as haploid insufficiency and could therefore be a possible mechanism contributing to a common phenotype of those with a deletion. Maternal disomy on the other hand would not result in

Table 6.1. Genetic differences between deletion Prader–Willi syndrome (PWS), disomy PWS, and normal

	Gene type		
	Maternally imprinted	Paternally imprinted	Non-imprinted
Deletion	Missing in PWS region; switched off elsewhere[a]	1 copy	1 copy in deleted region; 2 copies elsewhere
Disomy	Missing	2 copies	2 copies
Normal	1 copy	1 copy	2 copies

[a] Assuming all imprinted genes controlled from PWS/AS imprinting centre.

haploid insufficiency but in a double dose of any imprinted genes that are normally silenced in the paternally inherited homologue of chromosome 15 but which remain active in the maternal homologue, or complete lack of expression of any maternally imprinted gene located anywhere on chromosome 15, as both copies have the maternal imprint. These genes would include the Angelman syndrome gene *UBE3A* (which is paternally imprinted). There is still some debate as to whether the three GABA receptor genes β3, α5 and γ3, which lie within the distal Angelman syndrome part of the region are imprinted in the human brain or not, although in the mouse they are probably not.[4,5,6] The genetic differences between deletions, disomies and normal genetics are shown in Table 6.1.

From Table 6.1 it can be seen that differences between those without PWS and those with PWS due to chromosome 15 deletions or chromosome 15 disomies might be explained by different patterns of gene expression. For example, when people with PWS due to a chromosome 15 deletion or chromosome 15 disomy resemble one another but differ from people without PWS in some characteristic (i.e. the PWS phenotype), that characteristic is probably associated with the manifestations of maternally imprinted gene or genes in PWS at 15q11–q13 (PWS critical chromosomal region). Similarly, when people with PWS due to a deletion and those without PWS resemble one another but differ from people with PWS due to disomy on some characteristic, that characteristic is probably associated with the manifestations of paternally imprinted genes on chromosome 15. When people with PWS due to disomy and people without PWS resemble one another on some characteristic but differ from people with PWS due to a deletion, that characteristic is probably associated with the manifestations of having just one copy of a non-imprinted gene within the PWS critical region (the explanation of the fair for family skin/hair colouring observed in some with PWS due to deletions). This characterisation is perhaps simplistic and there are possible variations. For example, those with PWS due to isodisomies (as opposed to the common heterodisomy form of disomy) or those with deletions, which are atypically small or large in size, might also account for variations. These premises also assume that there is only one imprinting centre on chromosome 15, which appears to be the case, as extensive searches have failed to find another (E. B. Keverne, personal communication).

This chapter considers the characteristics associated with PWS, first, to see how people with PWS deletions and disomies differ, and second, with a view to classifying them into the three types of difference described earlier as, by doing so, this may give clues as to the genetic mechanisms associated with particular characteristics. Some characteristics are common to both PWS and other learning disabled groups (see Chapters 5, 7, 8) and therefore the aetiology of these characteristics are not confined to the genetics of chromosome 15.

Compared with the strong and wide ranging differences between people with PWS and people with normal genetics,[7,8,9,10] there are reports of very few and comparatively mild differences between the genetic subtypes. These reports are based on samples of the respective subtypes. However, these findings need to be backed up by repeat analysis as some of the differences may be a result of sampling error, as the cohorts studied were not representative samples. We acknowledge that our own work in this area is likely to be flawed in the same way because, although we started out with a population sample, we cannot guarantee that it was truly exhaustive and representative. Moreover, the number of people with disomies found was not large and the participants from outside the population area selectively contained a disproportionate number of people with the disomy form of PWS. The augmented sample therefore differed from the population sample in a number of ways and, for this reason, we have compared the genetic subtypes in the population samples where possible before using the augmented group for the analyses.

One interesting report,[10] which may well be due to sampling errors, based on 79 people with PWS due to disomy from seven different centres and 43 people with PWS due to deletions from two centres, found an excess of males in the disomy group (54) but not in the deletion group (19). However, when the disomies were classified as resulting from meiosis I, meiosis II or mitotic error, the male to female ratios were 41:18, 8:2 and 5:5, respectively. Further investigation appears to be warranted.

The PWS literature on deletion–disomy comparisons can be divided into five very general topic areas: differences at birth; differences in development; physical differences; cognitive differences; and behavioural differences. Among the former, the most commonly cited finding is increased maternal age in mothers of those with disomy PWS.[7,8,9] This has been ascribed to the mechanism of non-dysjunction responsible for disomies[11] (non-dysjunction is also the explanation of trisomy 21 in Down syndrome). Lower birth weight and body length at term, which are found in PWS compared with normal babies (although head circumference is normal), have not been found to differ consistently between genetic subtypes. Babies with PWS due to deletions had higher birth weight in one study[7] but lower in another,[8] and those babies with disomies had shorter birth length in one report[8] but not in the other.[7] These inconsistencies are probably due to sampling error, and researchers do not appear to have considered familial factors. Mean duration of gestation has not been found to differ between genetic subtypes.[8]

Differences in development include duration of feeding difficulties, age of onset of the food obsession and age at diagnosis of PWS. Apart from the former, usually measured as length of augmented feeding, the other two characteristics are by no means easy to determine. Mothers describe the transition, from the child with PWS being difficult to feed to actively seeking food, as a gradual process. Sometimes it took an outrageous food-eating episode to trigger the realisation, especially in children who were not diagnosed in infancy. On the other hand, as part of the Cambridge research, we were shown a video of a child of about seven months with disomy PWS being given a first chocolate finger biscuit and showing an excessive interest! Mothers often asked what we meant by 'age at diagnosis': age when they realised that their child had excessive eating and other behaviour problems (and did recognise or could have recognised PWS had they heard it described); age when someone suggested that their child had PWS; or age at which a formal diagnosis was made. The last was often long after the parents had taken measures to combat the worst symptoms and sometimes was only a formality. The articles in the literature do not explain which measure was used. Gunay-Aygun et al.[8] found no difference in length of augmented feeding or age of onset of hyperphagia, whereas Mitchell et al.[10] found that females with PWS due to disomy had shorter periods of such feeding and later onset of hyperphagia. The former study also found that mean age at diagnosis was higher in their disomy group, possibly because of diagnosis awaiting the onset of hyperphagia and behaviour problems.

The three characteristics that have been mentioned more than once in the literature as differences between the genetic subgroups are as follows: (1) an excess of 'fair for family' in those with deletions;[7,9,10] (2), fewer 'characteristic faces' in those with disomies;[9] and (3) fewer people with PWS due to disomies were thought to have a high pain threshold.[9] The excess of 'fair for family' in people with PWS due to deletions is one of the few differences to be given a full explanation. It is due to the fact that 15q11–q13 is the site for a non-imprinted gene with a recessive hypopigmentation allele. Those with deletions and those with isodisomy (as opposed to heterodisomy) are therefore more likely to express a recessive hypopigmentation gene either because of hemizygosity (i.e. only one copy – the other is absent because of the deletion), or because of homozygosity, as both copies of chromosome 15 are identical.

With respect to behavioural differences, the most consistent difference appears to be in self injurious behaviour, particularly skin picking.[9,12] Fewer people with PWS due to disomy have been reported to skin pick. In a questionnaire study of skin picking, Symons *et al.*[13] found that the most favoured sites were the front of the legs and the head and that people with PWS due to deletions picked at more sites than people with PWS due to disomies. However, this article was based on replies to questionnaires about skin picking mailed to parents of PWSA members and genetic subtype was based on parental report. Dykens *et al.*[12] compared 23 people with deletions with 23 age- and gender-matched people with PWS due to disomies on the Child Behaviour Checklist (CBC) and the Yale–Brown Obsessive–Compulsive Scales (Y-BOCS). Controlling for age and IQ, they found that those with PWS due to deletions scored more heavily on the CBC and on the Y-BOCS symptom-related distress. In particular, people with PWS due to deletions were more likely to skin pick, bite their nails, hoard, overeat, sulk and be withdrawn.

Cognitive differences between genetic subtypes have been mentioned in the literature from before the time that the disomy form was formally described. For example, Butler *et al.*[14] described differences between people with cytogenetic deletions and 'non-deletion' PWS (that is people with clinically diagnosed PWS but without a visible deletion in the PWS region) and found that those with a deletion had a lower mean IQ. A similar finding was reported by Dykens *et al.*[12] in their comparison of 23 pairs of age and gender matched subtypes. A study that looked at intellectual characteristics of 24 people with PWS due to deletions and 14 with disomies,[15] found no significant differences in overall IQ between the two groups but VIQ was significantly higher in the disomy group. Those with PWS due to disomies also had higher achievement scores. Cognitive profiles differed between the two groups with those with disomies doing significantly better on Information, Arithmetic, Vocabulary and Comprehension subscales, and those with deletions significantly better on Object Assembly. Visual recognition memory has been reported to be better in people with PWS due to disomies.[16] This finding was based on seven people with deletions, ten with disomies, and nine without PWS. Although the anecdotal evidence that people with PWS have particular skills with jigsaw puzzles has been around for a long time and was therefore included as a supportive item in the clinical diagnostic criteria, there have more recently been reports that this skill may apply only to people with the deletion subtype.[9,17]

Some of our own findings of subtype differences are presented in other chapters and we mention them here for completeness. In the chapter on medical conditions (Chapter 9), we look at reports of seizures and note that there were numbers of undiagnosed atypical episodes, comprising unexplained collapse, 'absences' or 'drooping'. It was noted that these episodes appeared more common in those individuals with maternal disomy of chromosome 15, 15/30 as compared with 10/57 of those with PWS due to a deletion.

In our investigation of cognition in PWS, described in Chapter 7, we found that the subtypes of the population sample did not differ on overall IQ (FSIQ) but differed on the two main subscales. Those with disomies scored about half a standard deviation higher on verbal intelligence (VIQ) and those with deletions higher by a similar amount on non-verbal intelligence (PIQ). There were two significant differences in cognitive profiles between the PWS subtypes, those with disomies scoring higher on the Vocabulary subscale and those with deletions higher on the Coding subscale (a measure of speed on a simple coding task). Significantly, the cognitive profiles of the learning disabled comparison group and the deletion PWS group were very similar, while that of the disomy PWS group was quite different. This pattern suggests the influence of a paternally imprinted gene (see Table 6.1).

The most striking finding from the Cambridge study was that relating to the prevalence of psychiatric disorder. One hundred per cent of those over age 28 years with PWS due to disomy and the one person with imprinting centre mutation had had a major psychiatric illness, while only one person with a deletion (11%), in that age group, had had such an illness. This latter rate is comparable to estimates for the learning disabled population (see Chapter 10).

The present report is based on all the people with PWS due to deletions or disomies in the augmented sample and those in the PWS-like comparison group described in Chapter 5. The 55 people with deletions had an age range from 0 to 46 years, including 25 under 18 years, the 30 with disomies had an age range from 0 to 46 years, including 17 under 18 years, and the 35 PWS-like group had an age range of 7 to 53 years, including 11 under 18 years. As described in Chapter 5, diagnostic criteria were scored on a three-point scale: strongly endorsed by informant; less strongly endorsed but present; and absent. Here the first two categories have been combined to give a present/absent dichotomy. The behavioural scorings have been similarly divided into present (that is, behaviour worse than the norm) and absent (behaviour no worse than the norm). Behaviour ratings of severity, taking account of both the extreme nature and frequency of occurrence, on a scale of 0 to 4 were recorded for the items in Section 4 of the PWS Questionnaire and a similar scale was constructed for eating behaviour, derived from the answers in Section 3 (Appendix 3.1).

Comparisons were made between PWS and PWS-like groups and also between the PWS subgroups, deletions and disomies. These comparisons showed that the genetic subgroups were not statistically different for the presence of any of our clinical criteria, but the PWS groups differed from the PWS-like group for the presence of *hypotonia, hypogonadism, feeding difficulties, small hands or feet, skin picking* and *obsessive–compulsive symptoms* (see also Chapter 5). Those with PWS due to

Table 6.2. Significant differences between Prader–Willi syndrome (PWS) deletion and disomy subgroups

Characteristic	Subjects	PWS deletion	PWS disomy	Significance
Possessiveness	All	33/49	24/26	0.05
	Adults	17/30	11/13	ns
	Children	16/19	13/13	ns
Sleep apnoea	All	6/49	10/26	0.01
	Adults	6/30	5/13	ns
	Children	0/19	5/13	ns
Eye problems	All	42/48	17/25	ns
	Adults	28/30	11/12	ns
	Children	14/18	6/13	0.01
High pain threshold	All	40/45	21/22	ns
	Adults	27/27	11/11	ns
	Children	13/18	10/11	0.05
Temperature regulation	All	25/41	16/23	ns
	Adults	13/23	11/12	0.05
	Children	12/18	5/11	ns
Jigsaw skills	All	26/46	5/23	ns
	Adults	16/28	2/10	0.05
	Children	10/18	3/13	ns

deletions or disomies were found to differ on the characteristics of *possessiveness, diagnosed sleep apnoea, eye problems* and *high pain threshold* in children, *poor temperature regulation* and *jigsaw skills* in adults, as shown in Table 6.2. They did not differ on average Body Mass Index in either adults (36.41 sp 13.04 v. 32.17 sp 8.47) or children (26.93 sp 10.76 v. 24.91 sp 6.45) nor in *daytime sleepiness scores* on the Epworth scale in adults (9.90 sp 5.07 v. 11.46 sp 5.19) or children (6.67 sp 3.68 v. 5.69 sp 3.33 in those with deletions or disomies, respectively). Severity of behaviour scores are shown in Table 6.3. Only three were significantly different for the two genetic subtypes and then only for the children, those with deletions being rated as more severe on *mood swings, stealing food,* and *severity of hyperphagia.*

At first sight it may appear counter-intuitive that children with deletions should have more severe (short-term) mood swings when it is adults with disomy PWS who exhibit a form of psychiatric disorder in which longer term mood changes drastically. However, in the chapter on behaviour (Chapter 8), our factor analysis of behaviours showed that mood swings were found to be part of the same factor as skin picking, which has previously been shown to be more common in those people with PWS due to deletions.[9, 13] See Chapter 8 for a possible genetic correlate.

Table 6.3. Comparison of severity of behaviour ratings between Prader–Willi syndrome (PWS) deletion and disomy subgroups

Behaviour	Subjects	PWS deletion	PWS disomy	Significance
Skin picking	Adults	2.97 (1.40)	2.77 (1.48)	
	Children	2.53 (1.61)	2.23 (1.92)	
Temper tantrums	Adults	3.07 (1.10)	3.00 (1.29)	
	Children	3.32 (0.89)	3.31 (1.25)	
Obsessional behaviour	Adults	3.21 (0.90)	3.31 (0.75)	
	Children	3.63 (0.68)	3.15 (0.90)	
Violent behaviour	Adults	2.21 (1.61)	2.00 (1.47)	
	Children	2.11 (1.45)	1.54 (1.51)	
Mood swings	Adults	1.59 (1.64)	1.62 (1.75)	
	Children	2.47 (1.61)	1.08 (1.75)	0.05
Argumentative	Adults	2.03 (1.50)	2.38 (1.61)	
	Children	2.16 (1.71)	1.38 (1.50)	
Lying	Adults	2.52 (1.55)	2.38 (1.39)	
	Children	1.67 (1.68)	0.92 (1.32)	
Stealing	Adults	2.82 (1.42)	2.62 (1.39)	
	Children	1.79 (1.72)	0.46 (0.78)	0.01
Hyperphagia	Adults	2.60 (0.62)	2.46 (0.78)	
	Children	2.00 (1.05)	1.38 (0.51)	0.05

Any differences between the genetic subtypes may have arisen entirely by chance, especially as our two groups are not necessarily representative of their respective genotypes. Therefore they will gain credibility if we can link them to the known genetic differences. We next consider how the genetic differences could have given rise to some of the observed phenotypic differences, through possible haploinsufficiency or possibly over or under-expression of imprinted genes, respectively. It is generally agreed that too little gene dosage is more detrimental than too much,[10] but it is difficult to reconcile this with the most striking difference yet found between the subtypes.

Possible haploinsufficiency

Eye problems were more frequent in children with a deletion than in those with disomy. The pink eye dilution gene (*OCA2*), a non-imprinted gene located within the Angelman syndrome region,[18] is present in a single copy in the deletion group, but in two copies in the maternal disomy group, which would make it a candidate for the observed differences. Another possible candidate gene, *TRPM1*, codes for

Table 6.4. Non-imprinted candidate haploinsufficiency genes in the Prader–Willi syndrome Angelman region

Gene symbol	Location	GDB	Unigene	Function
RNU66		10795819		Small nucleolar RNA
EHD4	15q11	10796174	Hs. 55058	GTPase
APBA2 (D15S1518E)		6277907	Hs. 26468	Amyloid β a4 precursor protein family a, member 2
NOLA3 (NOP10)	15q12		Hs. 14317	Nucleolar GAP protein family A, member 3
TRPM1	15q13q14	9837767	Hs. 43265	Transient receptor cation channel family M, member 1
LPHA		9958089	Hs. 202686	Member of the uteroglobin family
GCHFR	15q15	5195865	Hs. 83081	GTP cyclohydrolase regulatory protein
SLC12A6	15q13	9958559	Hs. 4876	KCl transporter family 12, member 6
PAK6	15q14	11501061	Hs. 21420	P21-activated protein kinase
SGNE1	15q11–q15	120376	Hs. 2265	Secretory granule neuroendocrine protein 1
OCA2	15q11.2–q12	136820		Oculocutaneous albinism type 2
TJP1	15q13	555860	Hs. 74614	Tight junction protein zo1
KIAA0013	D15S156–D15S165	9784280	Hs. 172652	Similar to GTPase-activating protein rhoGAP
CHRNA7	D15S156–D15S165	138751	Hs. 2540	Neuronal acetylcholine receptor protein α-7 chain precursor
MEIS2	15q13.3	9834323	Hs. 104105	Homeobox protein meis2

Note: The data in this Table were derived from different sources which were not always consistent, particularly with respect to gene order and location.

a transient cation channel expressed in the normal eye, which can also bind a micropthalamia-associated transcription factor.

Taking into account the severity of the respective behaviours, children with a PWS deletion were more affected by mood swings, stealing and hyperphagia. If any of these characteristics could be attributed to haploinsufficiency of non-imprinted genes, then several possible candidates are shown in Table 6.4. In addition, the imprinting status of the three GABA receptor genes, β3, α5, and γ3, which are known to lie within the Angelman syndrome region, is still not definitely established. The possible candidate genes include *SGNE1*, a secretory neuroendocrine protein active in the hypothalamus,[19] *CHRNA7*, a neuronal acetylcholine receptor protein which blocks neurotransmitter gated ion channels and *APBA2*, which is a member of a protein binding family found in the brain. The *APBA* gene family has been found to bind to the β-amyloid precursor protein and has been postulated to have a function in synaptic vesicle exocytosis. *KIAA0013* has a similar structure to the rhoGTPases, which are a family of small RAS-like GTPases that are involved in the inactivation of G proteins and so act in the signal transduction pathway. *NOLA3* or *NOP10* is a member of the small nucleolar RNP or snoRNP family A. *RNU66*, which is another member of the ACA box small nucleolar RNA gene group, is also located within the region. Small nucleolar RNA genes (snoRNAs), which are involved in pre-mRNA processing, have recently been described within the imprinting centre of the PWS region and have been implicated in presentation of the phenotype.[20, 21] MRG1 or MEIS2, found mainly in haemopoietic tissue and brain, belongs to the meis family of homeobox proteins and may be a transcription activator which is preferentially expressed in neonatal brain. The EHD4 or EH-domain containing protein 4 is implicated in nucleotide binding, while the GCHFR protein (p35) is a regulatory protein involved in the control of gtp cyclohydrolase activity.

Possible over/under expression of imprinted genes

A high pain threshold and diagnosed sleep apnoea were found to be more frequent in people with PWS due to chromosome 15 disomy. *ATP10C* is a paternally imprinted gene located within 15q11–q13, 200 kb distal to *UBE3A*. Both of these genes are ubiquitously expressed, particularly in the brain, and are subject to tissue-specific imprinting, and so either could be over-expressed in those with disomy.

Given the number of possible genetic differences between the subtypes of PWS, it is surprising that the two corresponding phenotypes have so few differences and yet so much in common. In particular, it is unusual that such a large excess or under expression of chromosomal material that would occur in those with disomies does apparently have such small effect. It is possible that as there is apparently no difference of expression of putatively important genes, the presence of two identical active imprinting centres within one cell could cause some material to become imprinted in a similar manner to the counting mechanism which operates in X-inactivation. Although the imprinting centres are believed to act only in *cis*, the spreading of X-inactivation also occurs in *cis* and the mechanism of imprinting is still unknown.

As will be apparent from the literature quoted in this chapter and from our findings presented here, similar findings are beginning to emerge from different samples of the two PWS subtypes. The most striking difference between the subtypes – rates of severe psychiatric disorder – was found because our original sample was a population sample. It is not yet clear whether or not such illness is inevitable in people with PWS due to disomy as they age, but confirmation of much higher rates in those with disomy compared to those with the deletion form of PWS has been received from researchers in several different countries (see Chapter 10). Some cognitive differences have also been demonstrated in several studies and appear to be real. Other differences found in our study need to be replicated. The research on genetic subtype differences is fairly recent, being dependent on reliable genetic diagnosis, and ideally there now needs to be cooperation between different centres to increase group sizes and so increase the reliability of the results. The implications of such findings are, however, important for both theoretical and practical reasons. In the case of the former, such differences are a measure of genetic influences on brain development. In the case of the latter, such findings may indicate the need for different approaches to, for example, education, and certainly the importance of an awareness of the risk of psychiatric illness, which can be difficult to diagnose but effectively treated, in those with disomy.

REFERENCES

1. Keverne, E. B. Genomic imprinting, maternal care, and brain evolution. *Hormones and Behaviour* **40** (2001), 146–155.
2. Haig, D. & Wharton, R. Prader-Willi syndrome and the evolution of human childhood. *American Journal of Human Biology* **15** (2003), 320–329.
3. Hall, J. G. Genomic imprinting: review and relevance to human diseases. *American Journal of Human Genetics* **46** (1990), 857–873.
4. LaSalle, J. M. & Lalande, M. Domain organisation of allele-specific replication within the GABRB3 gene cluster requires a biparental 15q11–13 contribution. *Nature Genetics* **9** (1995), 386–394.
5. Meguro, M., Mitsuya, K., Sui, H. *et al.* Evidence for uniparental, paternal expression of the human GABA receptor sub-unit genes, using microcell-mediated chromosome transfer. *Human Molecular Genetics* **6** (1997), 2127–2133.
6. Cassidy, S. B., Dykens, E. & Williams, C. A. Prader–Willi and Angelman syndromes: sister imprinted disorders. *American Journal of Medical Genetics* **97** (2000), 136–146.
7. Gillessen-Kaesbach, G., Robinson, W., Lohmann, D., Kaya-Westerloh, S., Passarge, E. & Horsthemke, B. Genotype–phenotype correlation in a series of 167 deletion and non-deletion patients with Prader–Willi syndrome. *Human Genetics* **96** (1995), 638–643.
8. Gunay-Aygun, M., Heeger, S., Schwartz, S. & Cassidy, S. B. Delayed diagnosis in patients with Prader–Willi syndrome due to maternal uniparental disomy 15. *American Journal of Medical Genetics* **71** (1997), 106–110.
9. Cassidy, S. B., Forsythe, M., Heeger, S. *et al.* Comparison of phenotype between patients with Prader–Willi syndrome due to deletion 15q and uniparental disomy 15. *American Journal of Medical Genetics* **68** (1997), 433–440.

10. Mitchell, J., Schinzel, A., Langlois, S. *et al.* Comparison of phenotype in uniparental disomy and deletion Prader–Willi syndrome: sex specific differences. *American Journal of Medical Genetics* **65** (1996), 133–136.

11. Ginsburg, C., Fokstuen, S. & Schinzel, A. The contribution of uniparental disomy to congenital development defects in children born to mothers at advanced child bearing age. *American Journal of Medical Genetics* **95** (2000), 454–460.

12. Dykens, E. M., Cassidy, S. B. & King, B. H. Maladaptive behavior differences in Prader–Willi syndrome due to paternal deletion versus maternal uniparental disomy. *American Journal on Mental Retardation* **104** (1999), 67–77.

13. Symons, F. J., Butler, M. G., Sanders, M. D., Feurer I. D. & Thompson, T. Self-injurious behavior and Prader–Willi syndrome: behavioral forms and body locations. *American Journal on Mental Retardation* **104** (1999), 260–269.

14. Butler, M. G., Meaney, F. J. & Palmer, C. G. Clinical and cytogenetic survey of 39 individuals with Prader–Labhart–Willi syndrome. *American Journal of Medical Genetics* **23** (1986), 793–809.

15. Roof, E., Stone, W., MacLean, W., Feurer, I. D., Thompson, T. & Butler, M. G. Intellectual characteristics of Prader–Willi syndrome: comparison of genetic subtypes. *Journal of Intellectual Disability Research* **44** (2000), 25–30.

16. Joseph, B., Egli, M., Sutcliffe, J. S. & Thompson, T. Possible dosage effect of maternally expressed genes on visual recognition memory in Prader–Willi syndrome. *American Journal of Medical Genetics* **105** (2001), 71–75.

17. Dykens, E. M. Are jigsaw puzzle skills 'spared' in people with Prader–Willi syndrome? *Journal of Child Psychology and Psychiatry* **43** (2002), 343–352.

18. Lee, S.-T., Nicholls, R. D., Bundey, S., Laxova, R., Musarella, M. & Spritz, R. A. Mutations of the P gene in oculocutaneous albinism, ocular albinism, and Prader–Willi syndrome plus albinism. *New England Journal of Medicine* **330** (1994), 529–534.

19. Gabreels, B. A., Swaab, D. F., de Kleijn, D. P. *et al.* Attenuation of the polypeptide 7B2, prohormone convertase PC2, and vasopressin in the hypothalamus of some Prader–Willi patients: indications for a processing defect. *Journal of Clinical Endocrinology and Metabolism* **83** (1998), 591–599.

20. Meguro, M., Mitsuya, K., Nomura, N. *et al.* Large-scale evaluation of imprinting status in the Prader–Willi syndrome region: an imprinted direct repeat cluster resembling small nucleolar RNA genes. *Human Molecular Genetics* **10** (2001), 383–394.

21. Runte, M., Huttenhofer, A., Gross, S., Kiefmann, M., Horsthemke, B. & Buiting, K. The IC-SNURF-SNRPN transcript serves as a host for multiple small nucleolar RNA species and as an antisense RNA for UBE3A. *Human Molecular Genetics* **10** (2001), 2687–2700.

7

Cognitive function and attainments

People with PWS frequently present with an apparently advanced level of vocabulary and conversational skills and thereby appear cognitively very able. Whilst this aspect of the development of people with PWS can be very positive, it can also have the significant disadvantage of raising expectations to a level that then results in high degrees of stress and failure. The anecdotes we give in this chapter help to illustrate this point as the particular problems or skills the anecdotes illustrate are not easily captured in a meaningful way through just reporting test scores. The rigidity of thinking of people with PWS and their inability to generalise can be very disabling, and can be associated with behaviour that can put the person at risk. For example, one mother of a daughter with PWS interviewed as part of the Cambridge study described how she had attempted to teach her daughter not to speak to strangers. The daughter could repeat the instructions and warnings she had been given and appeared to have understood, but the next day the mother found her daughter in their front garden accosting passers by with the question 'Are you a stranger?' Another much more common observation of this type was the teaching of kerb drill. The person with PWS could repeat and carry out at the kerb the drill they had been taught, but parents reported that they appeared unable to generalise this information to other situations and would ignore traffic and march straight out across the road at other locations. For these types of reasons there were several people with PWS seen as part of the study who were not allowed out unaccompanied.

People with PWS are good at dealing with concrete ideas but do not usually understand abstract concepts, although they will talk about them as if they understand. For example, when we asked parents or carers if the person they were supporting with PWS could recognise emotions, many said that they would recognise happiness and sadness if there was strong visible evidence (such as tears or smiles), but probably not other emotions. Time also seems to be a particular difficulty, not so much learning to tell the time, but rather appreciating the concept of the passage of time. For example, when people with PWS were asked if they visited relatives at least once a week almost none could give a reply that accorded with parent or carer.

If the question was rephrased to ask how many times in one week did they visit relatives, the reply could be out by several orders of magnitude.

Various other aspects of the cognitive function of people with PWS were observed as part of undertaking the cognitive assessment tests. Three people fell asleep in these sessions: daytime sleepiness is a feature of PWS and it seems to overtake the person with PWS very easily, particularly when in a situation he or she does not like or when he or she is thoroughly bored. Another frequent observation during the cognitive assessments was that, while taking part in the verbal tests, the person with PWS would answer an earlier question, or try to withdraw a previous answer. Similarly, people with PWS are supposed to have unusual skills with jigsaw puzzles, indeed this is one of the supportive diagnostic criteria, a common observation was that this presumed visuo-spatial skill was not usually evident in a related task, that of object assembly (a sub-test of the IQ test used). In this task, a cardboard representation of an object, divided by straight cuts into several pieces, is to be assembled as quickly as possible. There is no picture available but, as many people with PWS are said to be able to do jigsaws without a picture and even with the pieces blank side up, the absence of a picture should not prevent the completion of this task. However, advice given appeared frequently to be ignored and, for example, when the next piece tried clearly did not fit, all pieces were discarded.

One striking description frequently given by parents was the PWS child's capacity for imitation. Anecdotes included small children imitating their mother's polite enquiries to an acquaintance as to health, holidays and, even in one instance, blocked drains. Children with PWS were able to give recognisable impressions of TV personalities or to re-enact scenes they had seen on TV. On the other hand, it was apparent from both mothers' reports and during the assessment process that, for the person with PWS, generating new ideas for him or herself was very rare, even for those with IQ scores in the accepted normal range. The Comprehension Test in the Wechsler IQ battery asks questions about why we do certain things (Why do we cook certain types of food?) or have certain laws (Why are there laws about child employment?). Most people with PWS reply 'because it's the law', a few will give one response such as 'we cook food to stop it poisoning us', but it is extremely rare for any of them to generate a second reason for anything, however much encouragement is offered. One adult was found to have mastered two-column addition and subtraction, including 'carrying' and 'borrowing', which is fairly unusual in people with PWS. However, faced with a simple three-column addition, he was adamant that he could not do it because 'nobody showed me how to do those'. Arithmetic was observed to be a problem area for most people, with immature responses and strategies frequently observed. Many wanted things done for them, most counted on their fingers and found numbers above 10 difficult to manipulate, virtually none could 'add on' (that is, when adding two numbers, start from one of them and count on). Thus, there is a complexity to the cognitive strengths and weaknesses observed that is not apparent simply through the examination of cognitive test scores such as those given below.

It is generally found that people with PWS fall within the range of mild intellectual impairment: most having IQ scores in the range 50–75, but all having some indication of learning difficulties (cognitive deficits). A very few people with PWS have been described with IQs of over 100, but even with these people cognitive deficits were still apparent. For example, Sulzbacher, Crnic & Snow[1] refer to a 'P–W syndrome girl who has a tested IQ of over 100, but still appears to most casual observers as a mildly retarded person'. There was one young woman in our Cambridge study who tested with an IQ of 103 and who displayed cognitive deficits in short-term memory and comprehension, particularly of abstract concepts.

At the other extreme, a few people have IQs of less than 40, but our experience suggests that they may have sustained neurological damage in addition to having PWS. This would not be surprising, given the abnormal presentations of some babies with PWS at birth and the long labours experienced by many mothers. In the Cambridge population sample, only one-third (18 of 54 mothers questioned) were said to have had a normal delivery when their child with PWS was born. Twelve of the 54 were breech presentations, half of which were delivered by Caesarian section. In addition, 25% were more than one month premature, and 20% were two or more weeks late.

Cognitive functioning and genetics

In the non-learning-disabled population, general ability is influenced both by genetic and environmental factors with the genetic component estimated as accounting for between 0.50 and 0.80 of the variance, and being mediated by many genes.[2] Human cognition is supposed to be made up of a general ability, common to all aspects, and many specific abilities. A large number of genes must contribute to human cognition, as evidenced by cognitive variations between individuals, and we might suppose that some contribute to general ability and others to specific abilities. It is not then so surprising how devastating the effects of certain single gene defects can be on the whole of cognition, while the effects of other differences in genotype can be quite subtle, affecting only specific aspects.

For those genetic syndromes associated with early developmental delay and learning disabilities, such as PWS, it is assumed that the gene(s) associated with the syndrome are expressed in the developing brain in normal people, and that it is the failure of expression of these gene(s) in those with PWS that leads to abnormal brain development, and thus impaired cognitive, emotional and/or social development. Currently, the particular abnormal developmental processes leading to the learning disabilities, the patterns of general ability and the factors that influence the extent of variation in the degree of severity associated with different syndromes are often unknown.

The study of genetic syndromes associated with learning disabilities can give information about the genetic component of cognition. Potentially important pointers to the nature of the genetic influences on cognition include the distribution and heritability of general ability in people with a given syndrome and the systematic differences in profiles of abilities between people with different syndromes, especially when a specific ability or disability is associated with a particular syndrome. In PWS there is also the possibility that those with the different genetic subtypes differ in general ability and/or in the profile of abilities. Ideally, such investigations require representative samples (or repeated random sampling) of those with the syndrome. For many genetic syndromes, such population-based cohorts have not been obtained.

Cognitive functioning in people with PWS: previous literature

The literature on cognitive functioning and achievement in PWS is somewhat mixed in the findings. People with PWS have been variously described as having 'usually mild to moderate mental retardation', 'normal intelligence in a significant number of cases', 'learning disabilities', 'characteristic cognitive weaknesses', 'good reading skills', and 'weakness in arithmetic skills'. It is not always possible to deduce from the text on what basis these claims have been made. Generally, the first two are based on the results of an IQ test indicating that IQ is usually found to be in the ranges 50–70 or 50–85[3,4] and as many as one-quarter (or one-fifth) have an IQ over 70 (or over 80, depending on the rating system used).[3,4] The other descriptions are usually based on discrepancies between IQ subscale scores or on the findings from educational attainment tests.[5,6] In the UK, the term 'learning disabilities' (equivalent to the term 'mental retardation') refers to a global lowering of ability scores in the context of early developmental delay, whereas 'specific learning difficulties' refers to conditions such as dyslexia and dyscalculia, in which specific areas of ability are affected, resulting in particular areas of attainment being abnormally low in relation to general levels of IQ and other attainments. The evidence indicates that in PWS there is both a global lowering of ability and possibly more specific cognitive disabilities.

Reports of cognitive functioning in people with PWS have suffered from methodological drawbacks. First, they have usually been based on volunteer or clinical samples of people with PWS, and no attempt has been made to assess the representativeness of such samples. Second, early reports in particular (some based on clinical criteria and some on visible deletions only) may have misclassified individuals as having PWS. Experience from our Cambridge study indicates that prior to the establishment of genetic criteria a proportion of all 'cases' were misclassified. These drawbacks may explain the discrepancies and contradictions within the literature. However, some findings have been replicated in samples of people with genetic confirmation of PWS, and a meta-analysis of 56 studies has been published.[4] It is now generally accepted that, as a group, people with PWS perform better on visuo-spatial tasks, have poor short-term memories, deficits in sequential processing, poor socialisation skills, and exceptional skills with jigsaw puzzles.[6,7,8] It has also been reported that IQ is not related to weight and does not decline with age.[6]

Since the two main categories of genetic abnormality in PWS were established, comparisons of cognitive performance between people in the deletion and disomy subgroups have been described. Roof *et al.*[9] found that people with disomies had a higher average verbal intelligence (VIQ), whereas there was no significant difference in average performance, or non-verbal intelligence (PIQ). In an analysis of subscale scores, they found that most verbal subscale mean scores were higher for those with disomies, whereas the mean Object Assembly subscale score was higher for those with deletions.

In contrast with the usual emphasis on disability, the consensus diagnostic criteria contain a 'supportive' item: unusual skill with jigsaw puzzles. Dykens *et al.*[10] conducted an investigation using three groups of children: a group with PWS; an IQ-matched learning disabilities (LD) group; and an age-matched normal group. Each child was tested on a jigsaw puzzle task (how many pieces could be correctly placed in three minutes), a word-search task, and also the block design and object assembly subtests from the WISC.[11] For all tests other than the jigsaw puzzle, the mean scores of the three groups were in the order: normal > PWS > LD; for the jigsaw test, the order was PWS > normal > LD. On dividing the PWS group into those with deletions and those with disomies, the exceptional performance with the jigsaw was found to hold only for the deletion group. Dykens *et al.*[10] concluded that PWS due to chromosome 15 deletions is associated with an exceptional skill. Our findings were not consistent with this observation (see below).

The Cambridge study of cognition

In our Cambridge study we asked what mechanism(s) might account for the distribution of general ability in the PWS population sample, and whether there are systematic cognitive differences between genetic subtypes and, if so, what these differences tell us about genetic influences on cognition, and what implications (if any) this might have for understanding cognitive development in the general population. We also investigated the extent to which the data supported the presence of an exceptional skill (jigsaw puzzles) in those with the deletion subtype of PWS. Psychometrically, we looked at general ability, ability profiles, and attainment in reading, spelling, and arithmetic abilities in people with PWS, for both the population-based sample and the augmented sample, and compared the findings with published norms and with those of a learning disabled group of mixed aetiology. We looked at correlations with age and Body Mass Index (BMI) for any systematic influences on cognition and compared ability profiles of those in the deletion, disomy, and the LD groups. Our hypothesis was that there would be a global downward shift in Full Scale IQ of a similar degree in those with PWS due to chromosome 15 disomies and chromosome 15 deletions, but that there would be specific differences in cognitive profiles between the two subtypes reflecting subtly different genetic influences on brain development.

As indicated in Chapter 3, cognitive abilities were assessed in people with PWS, over age three years, by the age-appropriate Wechsler Intelligence Scales.[11] The few people with PWS of very low IQ could not be accurately assessed, since the scales have a cut-off level of 45 on both the verbal and performance scales. Anyone scoring below the cut-off level of 45 on the verbal (*VIQ*), performance (*PIQ*), and full-scale (*FSIQ*) of the Wechsler IQ tests was given a score of 40. In some analyses (clearly indicated in text or tables) these low scorers were excluded. A very small minority of people (three PWS and seven LD) in the study either found it difficult to fully co-operate or had physical disabilities that prevented administration of some test items. Under these circumstances, pro-rated totals were used to calculate full-scale IQ, as provided in the relevant manuals. To compare relative strengths and weaknesses in cognitive profiles, for each individual a relative subtest score was calculated as follows:

[scaled score on given subtest x100]/[average scaled score on all subtests].

Gender differences in mean *FSIQ, VIQ, PIQ,* and in relative subtest scores were investigated in the augmented PWS group and between the genetic subtypes.

There were no significant gender differences in mean *FSIQ, VIQ, PIQ,* or in relative subtest scores in the augmented PWS group, or for those in the separate deletion and disomy groups (*t*-tests, $p = .05$). Table 7.1 shows the means and standard deviations of *age, FSIQ, VIQ, PIQ, attainment in reading, spelling* and *arithmetic,* and current *BMI* for the population PWS sample, the full PWS sample, and the comparison LD sample. Table 7.2 shows the means and standard deviations of the same set of variables for the main genetic subtypes (i.e., deletions and disomies) of PWS. Table 7.2 is based on the subset of the full PWS sample for which genetic subtype was established.

Histograms of frequency distributions for *FSIQ, reading, spelling,* and *arithmetic standard scores* are shown in Figures 7.1 to 7.4 for the population sample, the augmented sample, and the comparison LD group. The distribution of IQ is approximately normal for the population-based group of people with PWS, but

Table 7.1. Means, ranges and standard deviations of age, full-scale IQ, verbal IQ, performance IQ, current BMI and attainments for the three groups: population sample Prader–Willi syndrome (Pop. PWS), all PWS, and Learning disabilities (LD)

	Pop. PWS		All PWS		LD	
	All IQ	IQ > 40	All IQ	IQ > 40	All IQ	IQ > 40
Age: mean	20.9	21.0	20.4	20.3	21.2	21.1
range	4–46	4–46	4–46	4–46	5–49	5–49
SD	12.1	12.4	10.9	11.1	14.1	14.2
n	58	52	96	88	36	31
FSIQ: mean	61.4	62.6	63.5	64.3	63.4	66.4
range	40–103	45–103	40–103	45–103	40–99	41–99
SD	13.0	12.2	11.7	11.0	16.6	15.2
n	55	52	91	88	35	31
VIQ: mean	63.8	65.1	66.8	67.7	64.5	67.7
range	40–101	46–101	40–101	46–101	40–101	46–101
SD	13.3	12.3	12.4	11.6	16.5	14.8
n	55	52	91	88	35	31
PIQ: mean	63.1	64.4	64.0	64.8	66.5	69.9
range	40–105	40–105	40–105	40–105	40–105	45–105
SD	12.9	12.0	11.3	10.6	17.5	15.6
n	55	52	91	88	35	31
BMI: mean	33.2	33.2	31.5	31.7	29.1	28.7
range	16–76	16–76	16–76	16–76	15–56	16–54
SD	12.2	12.5	11.4	11.5	10.4	9.6
n	53	49	91	85	34	29
Reading[b]: mean	57.2	59.1	62.9	64.2	54.8	58.8
range	20–104	20–104	20–106	20–106	20–91	20–91
SD	28.0	27.7	27.1	26.7	22.3	19.9
n	48	45	80	77	29	26
Spelling[b]: mean	54.3	56.6	60.1	61.7	53.0	56.8
range	20–103	20–103	20–110	20–110	20–86	20–86
SD	26.1	25.3	25.1	24.3	20.8	18.3
n	48	45	80	77	29	26
Arith.[b]: mean	47.5	49.4	53.1	54.4	52.6	56.4
range	20–90	20–90	20–96	20–96	20–94	20–94
SD	23.6	23.3	22.8	22.3	25.7	24.4
n	48	45	80	77	29	26
Reading[b]: undmean		4.9		3.7		12.7
Spelling[b]: undmean		11.8		10.6		16.3
Arith.[b]: undmean		13.8		12.7		12.9

[a] Includes only those with any cognitive data, i.e. ages greater than three years.

[b] Ages eight years and above.

Undmean: mean under-achievement.

Table 7.2. Means, ranges and standard deviations of age, full-scale IQ (FSIQ), verbal IQ (VIQ), performance IQ (PIQ), attainments in reading, spelling and arithmetic for the genetic subtypes deletions, and disomies for the population Prader–Willi syndrome (PWS) and all PWS (all IQ)[a]

	Deletion PWS (IQ > 40)		Disomy PWS (IQ > 40)	
	All	Pop	All	Pop
Age: mean	21.7	21.2	18.4	24.6
range	5–46	5–46	4–46	6–46
SD	11.4	13.2	12.4	14.7
n	46	28	25	11
FSIQ: mean	63.8	61.6	63.3	62.9
range	46–91	46–91	46–82	46–82
SD	10.2	11.2	9.7	10.4
n	46	28	25	11
VIQ: mean	65.8	62.4	69.7	68.8
range	46–91	46–91	50–95	50–93
SD	10.6	11.0	11.6	11.6
n	46	28	25	11
PIQ: mean	65.9	65.6	61.05	60.3
range	47–94	47–94	40–79	40–73
SD	9.5	10.8	8.7	9.7
n	46	28	25	11
Reading: mean	60.2	55.6	71.3	64.7
range	20–103	20–103	20–106	20–104
SD	26.7	27.0	26.7	28.7
n	41	24	21	10
Spelling: mean	59.2	53.8	66.8	60.6
range	20–96	20–96	20–110	20–103
SD	24.0	24.4	24.6	25.7
n	41	24	21	10
Arith.: mean	54.4	51.1	53.5	45.9
range	20–86	20–86	20–90	20–90
SD	21.0	22.8	23.7	24.6
n	41	24	21	10
BMI: mean	33.3	34.6	28.5	30.8
range	16–76	16–76	16–50	21–50
SD	13.0	14.6	8.4	8.7
n	45	27	25	11

[a] Includes only those with any cognitive data, i.e. ages greater than three years.
BMI: Body Mass Index.

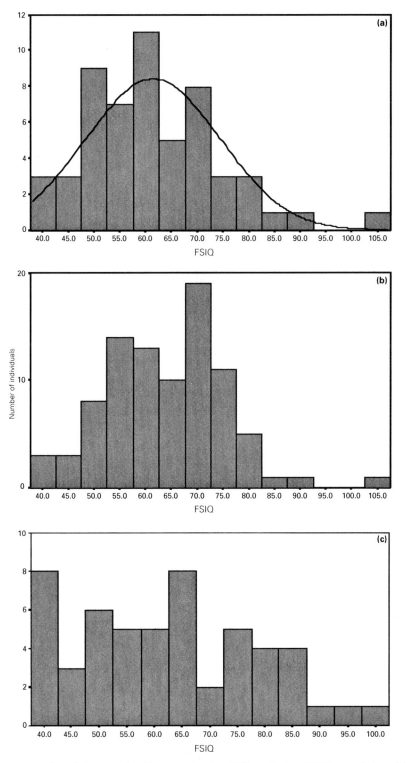

Figure 7.1. Frequencies of IQ scores for (a) $n = 55$ Prader–Willi syndrome (PWS) population; (b) $n = 93$ all PWS; and (c) $n = 54$ learning disabilities group. FSIQ: full scale IQ.

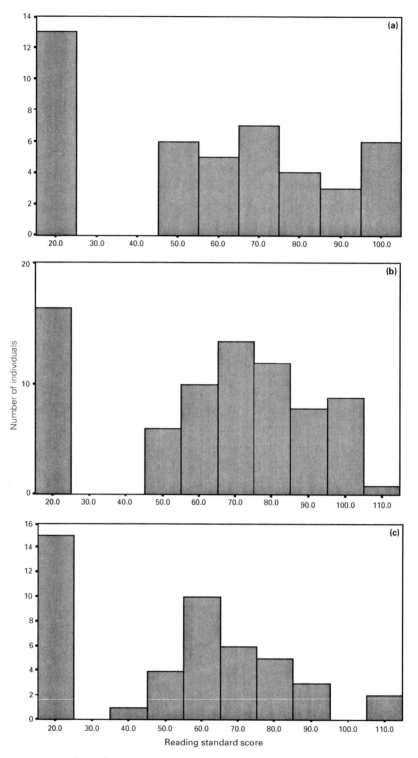

Figure 7.2. Frequencies of Reading attainment standard scores for (a) $n = 48$ Prader–Willi syndrome (PWS) population; (b) $n = 81$ all PWS; (c) $n = 47$ learning disabilities group.

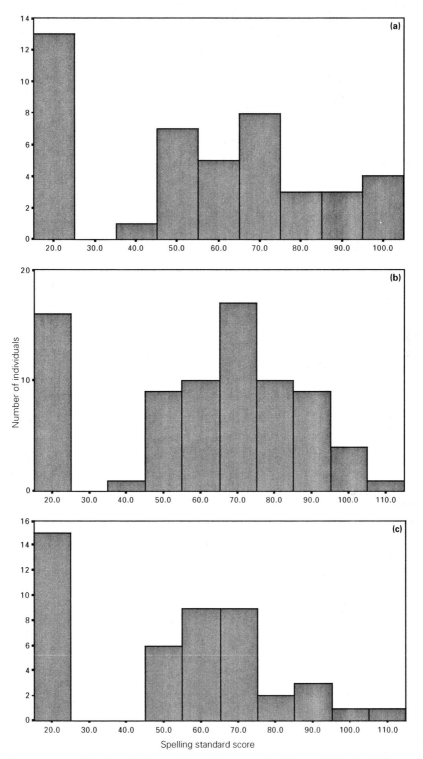

Figure 7.3. Frequencies of Spelling attainment standard scores for (a) $n = 48$ Prader–Willi syndrome (PWS) population; (b) $n = 81$ all PWS; (c) $n = 47$ learning disabilities group.

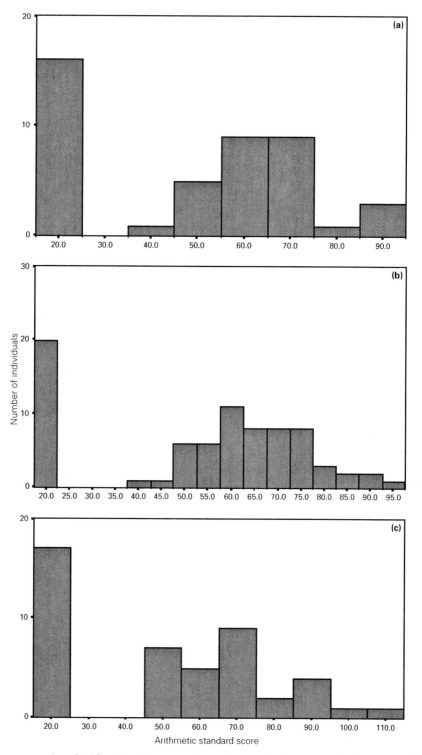

Figure 7.4. Frequencies of Arithmetic attainment standard scores for (a) $n = 48$ Prader–Willi syndrome (PWS) population; (b) $n = 81$ all PWS; (c) $n = 47$ learning disabilities group.

not for the LD group. The augmented PWS group also has a different IQ distribution, which we propose is a consequence of selection bias. The scatter plots (Figure 7.5) of achievement (*reading, spelling, and arithmetic*) against IQ show that, for both children and adults, the variations in underachievement are wide. This will be considered further below.

Correlations of *age* and *BMI* with *FSIQ* and the subscales *VIQ* and *PIQ* and all subtests for the population PWS and for deletion and disomy population groups, when corrected for the number of tests, were all non-significant.[6] This agrees with the previous literature.[7]

There were no statistically significant differences in mean standard scores on the subtests of the Wechsler Ability scales for the PWS population sample, the PWS augmented sample, and the LD group, or between the population sample and the augmented sample for the two PWS genetic subtypes.[6]

Figure 7.6 compares the cognitive profiles (relative scores computed as already described above) of three groups: the LD group and the two genetic subtypes of PWS. It can be seen that those in the deletion and LD groups are quite similar, while those in the disomy group differ from both. Those with disomies have a cognitive strength, relative to the other two groups, in *vocabulary* ($P = 0.001$), and a cognitive weakness in *coding* (speed) ($P = 0.01$).

Jigsaw puzzle skills

In order to investigate the reported skills with jigsaw puzzles we compared the means and standard deviations of the *FSIQ, VIQ, PIQ,* and certain Wechsler Ability subscale scores across five groups: (1) those with deletions reported by an informant to have exceptional skills with jigsaw puzzles; (2) those with deletions said not to have exceptional skills with jigsaw puzzles; (3) those with disomies said to have exceptional skills with jigsaw puzzles; (4) those with disomies said not to have exceptional skills with jigsaw puzzles; and (5) those with learning disabilities not due to PWS. None of this last group was said by mothers to have exceptional skill with jigsaw puzzles (see Table 7.3). In all groups, those people in which informants said the person had some skill, but it was not exceptional, were omitted for the purposes of this analysis. Our data suggested that not all those people with PWS due to deletions have similar elevated visuo-spatial skills, but that visuo-spatial abilities is an area of relative strength in those people with reported jigsaw puzzle skills. However, strikingly, even these people were surpassed on the *Object Assembly* subtest by the IQ matched LD group. This is a surprising result if exceptional jigsaw puzzle skills are innate in those with this PWS genetic subtype and suggests that a combination of some innate ability and repeat practice may be the explanation.

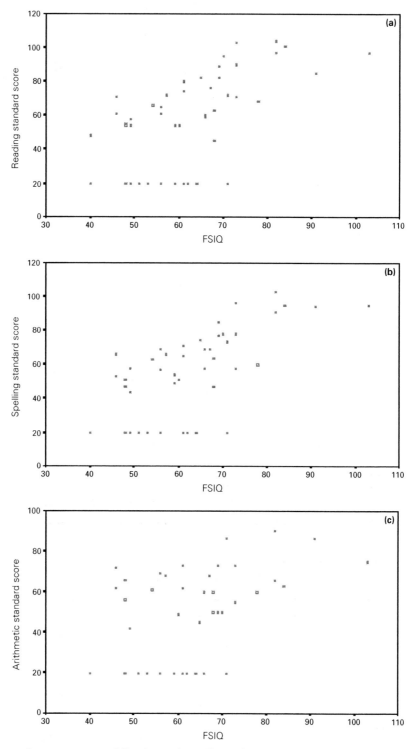

Figure 7.5. Attainments versus ability in Prader–Willi syndrome population sample: (a) Reading; (b) Spelling; (c) Arithmetic. FSIQ: full scale IQ.

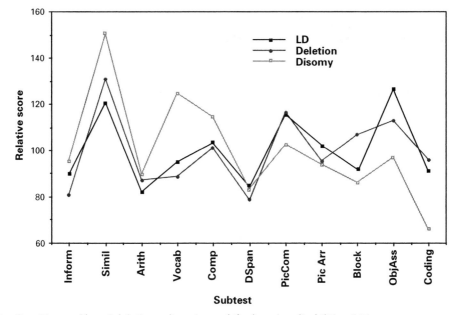

Figure 7.6.   Cognitive profiles of deletions, disomies and the learning disabilities (LD) group.

Conclusions on the cognitive abilities of people with PWS

The Cambridge study was the first population-based study of the cognitive abilities and attainments of children and adults with the genetically determined PWS. As hypothesised, and in keeping with previous reports, we found a marked downward shift in global ability, regardless of genetic subtype, together with subtle specific cognitive differences between those with deletions and those with disomy. Five people over age three years included in our population study did not wish to participate in the cognitive testing; parental and carer reports would put them in the 50–80 FSIQ range. Three people with PWS and seven in the LD group scored below the Wechsler scale floor on both VIQ and PIQ. As the relevant tables show, including these participants by assigning them an IQ score of 40 or omitting them, makes little difference to the results. Thus, we conclude that those in this sample are representative of the range of abilities and attainments found in people with PWS.

The finding of a near normal distribution of FSIQ scores for the PWS population suggests that one effect of the PWS genotype may be to shift the ability distribution downwards by about 40 IQ points. The fact that all ability subscales are affected, points to a global, rather than a specific effect on cognition. The question of whether this is a systematic (roughly the same for each individual) or a random effect (varying unsystematically between individuals) requires familial studies, and an estimate

Table 7.3. Cognitive performances of groups of deletion (Del), disomy (Dis), and learning disabilities (LD) subtypes said to have, or lack, respectively, skills with jigsaw puzzles

	Del-Yes $n=18$	Del-No $n=18$	Dis-Yes $n=2$	Dis-No $n=18$	LD (No) $n=39$
Age	25.2	20.6	16.0	15.9	23.2
BMI	35.3	34.1	44.2	26.8	29.6
FSIQ	65.8	62.3	60.5	63.7	65.8
VIQ	65.9	66.4	62.0	71.3	67.9
PIQ	69.9	61.9	64.0	60.8	68.6
Mean scaled and relative subtest scores					
Information	3.1	3.5	1.5	4.4	4.2
	68.8	88.6	42.2	102.7	89.0
Similarities	5.7	5.7	6.0	6.1	5.4
	136.1	141.1	174.3	156.4	123.9
Arithmetic	3.2	3.4	3.0	4.1	3.6
	74.5	89.0	78.9	93.0	81.0
Vocabulary	3.8	4.0	2.5	5.3	4.3
	83.3	100.0	66.6	131.2	98.4
Comprehension	4.2	4.4	3.0	5.0	4.6
	97.1	106.8	78.9	116.9	106.5
Digit span	2.9	3.4	1.0	3.6	4.1
	64.2	89.6	30.0	84.9	80.5
Picture completion	4.7	4.4	4.0	4.0	4.8
	110.0	119.2	125.4	99.1	114.7
Picture arrangement	3.9	4.0	5.0	3.6	4.6
	89.8	100.8	149.8	81.4	104.8
Block design	5.7	3.1	3.5	3.5	4.2
	136.5	77.8	102.1	78.6	89.5
Object assembly	5.2	3.2	6.5	3.6	5.4
	136.4	84.7	197.5	89.0	123.9
Coding	4.3	4.0	2.0	3.1	4.0
	97.4	95.1	54.4	69.1	91.8

BMI: Body Mass Index; FSIQ: full scale IQ; VIQ: verbal IQ; PIQ: performance IQ.

of heritability of general ability in the PWS population. Some support for a systematic effect comes from a recent study of correlations with maternal IQ.[13] This global effect occurs regardless of the specific PWS genotype and therefore we propose that there is likely to be a single mechanism having a direct and specific effect on brain development consequent upon the absence of expression of an imprinted gene. Neither the actual gene that might have this effect nor the underlying pathophysiological mechanism is known at present. We consider this further in Chapter 12. Mild cortical atrophy and a small brainstem have been reported and a reduced neurone count in the brains of people with PWS has been hypothesised.[14]

Our findings support the reports of cognitive differences between those in the deletion or disomy genetic subgroups,[9, 15] although some of the reported differences may be due to the sampling methods used. We have found higher verbal abilities in those with chromosome 15 disomies (and our results also suggest lower performance abilities), while those with deletions are similar to our general LD group. A new finding is that the disomy group have particular difficulty with *coding*, and score very poorly on that subtest.

Although exceptional skill with jigsaw puzzles has become one of the supportive criteria in the clinical diagnosis of PWS, our findings suggested that the observed effect could be equally well explained on the basis of prior practice. Indeed, given the PWS compulsiveness to repetitive behaviour (especially for word-search tasks and jigsaw puzzles), it seems likely that practice in the PWS group would far exceed that in either of the other groups. Our findings with regard to the two WISC subtests of *block design* and *object assembly*, show that our PWS group had lower scores than the LD group and far below the average for the general population. However, those with deletions certainly did better than those with disomies (but still no better than the LD group). On dividing the PWS groups according to mothers' (or main carers') reports of exceptional skills with jigsaws, people with deletions said to have such skills were found to perform better on these two WISC subtests. Our interpretation of Dykens *et al.*'s[10] findings is that there may be a practice effect (carers had noticed their charges doing jigsaws on many occasions), but that their initial interest in such puzzles may arise from a natural relative ability in these aspects of visuo-spatial function that is predominately present in those with deletions.

Overall the IQ profile of those with disomy is different from those with deletion, and from the LD comparison group. Within each genetic group, we expect individual cognitive profiles to vary, as they do in the general population, due to individual genotypic differences, but the consistent difference between genetic subtypes suggests the influence of either over or under expression of a specific maternally or paternally expressed gene on chromosome 15 (see Chapter 6). The two genetic subtypes could have a different pattern of expression of maternally imprinted genes located outside the PWS critical chromosomal region, and of paternally expressed genes located either inside or outside this region. We therefore hypothesise not only that failure of expression of a PWS specific gene accounts for the much lower mean full scale IQ score in all people with PWS, but that there are also more subtle effects on brain function and on cognitive performance, which is characterised as a better verbal performance for those with disomy, and better visuo-spatial performance for at least some with deletions. In our study there were no significant gender effects known to influence the profile of cognitive abilities, either in the PWS group as a whole or in the genetic subtypes investigated, but we hypothesise that there may be genetic effects on cerebral lateralisation that could account for these cognitive differences between genetic subtypes. Further studies need to investigate the influence of parental cognitive abilities, sex hormone levels, and other measures of cerebral dominance to try and elucidate further whether such a hypothesis can be sustained or not.

Achievement and underachievement in PWS

The old belief that all people with learning disabilities go through the same intellectual, cognitive and emotional development and require the same curriculum and teaching methods is now being challenged. Current opinion is that the particular cause of a person's learning disability may have a specific and characteristic influence on the development of that child.[16] In turn these patterns of cognitive, linguistic and behavioural strengths and weakness may affect the learning potential and ultimate attainment of that person. For example, the literature on achievement by people with PWS generally reports that they have 'good reading skills' and 'weakness in arithmetic skills'. Understanding the individual and his or her unique attributes, together with knowledge of the impact that a specific disorder has on his or her development, may provide a guide to the best form of education for that individual.

The Cambridge study of underachievement in PWS

We explored the level of attainment in a cohort of people with PWS compared to people with LD due to other causes. The aims of this part of the study were to investigate the extent to which people with PWS reached the attainments predicted by their IQ, and to investigate factors that might be associated with any underachievement.

As indicated in Chapter 3, attainments were measured by the three Wechsler test batteries WORD, WOND and WOLD[17, 18] for ages 8 to 16, and by the WRAT[19] for ages 17 and above. People who failed to reach a standard score of 45, the lower limit of the tests, were given a token score of 20. They were excluded from the discriminant analyses.

The manuals for the Wechsler achievement tests each give a table of expected standard scores on the test predicted from the full-scale IQ score on the WISC-lll. The manual for the WRAT-3 gives means and standard deviations for scores of the standardisation sample on the WAIS-R and the three attainment subscales and

Table 7.4. Regression equations of attainment measures on full-scale IQ

Attainment measure	Regression equation
WORD reading	$P(\text{reading}) = 40 + 0.6 * \text{FSIQ}$
WORD spelling	$P(\text{spelling}) = 50 + 0.5 * \text{FSIQ}$
WOND arithmetic	$P(\text{arithmetic}) = 42.5 + 0.575 * \text{FSIQ}$
WRAT3 reading	$P(\text{reading}) = 51.8 + 0.424 * \text{FSIQ}$
WRAT3 spelling	$P(\text{spelling}) = 50 + 0.446 * \text{FSIQ}$
WRAT3 arithmetic	$P(\text{arithmetic}) = 37.5 + 0.559 * \text{FSIQ}$

correlations between them. Separate regression equations of attainment in reading, spelling and arithmetic on IQ for each of the two age groups were calculated from the above information and used to predict attainment scores from full-scale IQ scores. Actual attainment scores were subtracted from predicted scores to give the degree of underachievement (in standard score units). Underachievement was defined only for IQ scores greater than 40 and for attainment standard scores above 44. Table 7.4 gives the regression equations for attainment (reading, spelling, arithmetic) on full-scale IQ score as derived for the respective standardisation samples of the Wechsler and WRAT-3 attainment tests. Using these to predict attainment scores from IQ scores, underachievement was calculated as predicted score minus actual score for each of reading, spelling and arithmetic.

Scatterplots of IQ against achievement, for those in the augmented PWS and LD groups respectively, are presented in Figure 7.5 and show that there were wide variations in (under)achievement for both groups. Mean underachievement varied by academic domain and by group. This is shown in Figure 7.7 where underachievement in reading and, to a lesser extent, spelling is smaller, but underachievement in mathematics is similar in the PWS and LD groups.

Possible explanatory variables for underachievement are detailed below. Measures that were available in this study are indicated in italics. Ethical considerations, non-availability of information and subjectivity of information precluded such possibly relevant variables as family circumstances, teaching methods and styles, certain personality traits, self-esteem and measures of motivation. Children with PWS often have severe behavioural problems such as stealing food or money, immature social behaviour, temper tantrums and obsessive–compulsive behaviour (*Aberrant Behaviour Checklist scores* and *Vineland: Socialisation Domain standard score*). Because of the above behaviours, mainstream schools may be unable to cope and such children may be placed in special needs schools where there are more staff available, despite the fact that the person with PWS may have the ability to cope

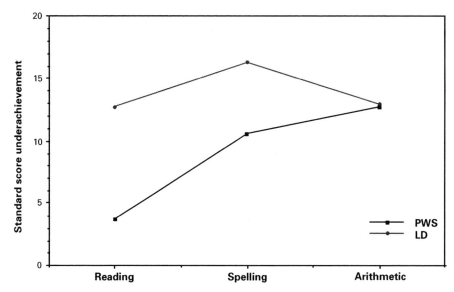

Figure 7.7. Mean Underachievement of Prader–Willi syndrome (PWS) and learning disabilities (LD) groups across academic domains.

with the academic demands of mainstream school. Emphasis in special schools is often placed on the practical skills of coping with personal needs, domestic tasks and community rules (*Percentage of schooling, to date, spent in special needs schools; Vineland: Daily Living Skills Domain standard score*). Children with PWS are very demanding of parents: repetitive questioning and demands for inflexible routines being the most onerous for the majority of those we interviewed. Larger families might be expected to decrease the amount of parental attention available to a child with the syndrome (*Number of siblings*). People with PWS have a preoccupation with food and seem to spend a great deal of time thinking about it; this could be a distraction from their academic studies (*severity of eating disturbance, BMI*). Daytime sleepiness (witnessed in some cases by falling asleep during our assessments!) is one of the minor clinical criteria for PWS (*Score on Epworth Sleepiness Scale*). Normal children often underachieve because of such neurological disorders as attention deficit, hyperactivity or autism (*screens for ADD, HD and autistic traits*).

Given some of the specific characteristics of people with PWS, we hypothesised that severe behavioural problems, problematic food related behaviours, immature social behaviour and aberrant behaviours such as temper tantrums and obsessive–compulsive behaviour may all influence the level of attainment, and therefore we have included measures of these variables, which were systematically assessed as part of the phenotypic study. Despite relatively mild intellectual impairments, we noted that many people with PWS had been educated at special needs schools. The type of approach in special school described earlier may not in itself maximise educational skills and therefore we have included '*percentage of schooling (to date) spent in special needs schools*' as a variable. Other variables, which we predicted might affect attainment levels in those with PWS or those in the comparison group, included *family size*, daytime sleepiness (as measured by *scores on the Epworth sleepiness scale*), *attention deficit, hyperactivity* and *autistic traits* screen scores.

Table 7.1 shows the means and standard deviations of *age, current BMI, full-scale IQ, verbal IQ, performance IQ, attainments in reading, spelling and arithmetic, and underachievements in reading, spelling and arithmetic* for the population PWS sample, the full PWS sample and the comparison LD sample.

For the full PWS group and for the LD group, correlations of underachievement (defined above) in reading, spelling and arithmetic, and the influence of the variables listed below, were examined. These variables were also entered in multiple regression analyses as explanatory variables with *degree of underachievement* as the dependent variable. The variables examined were: *age; gender; genetic subtype; number of siblings; autistic traits screen score; attention deficit screen score; hyperactivity screen score; aberrant behaviour score; body mass index; severity of eating abnormality; daytime sleepiness score; Vineland Daily Living Skills domain standard score; Vineland Socialisation Domain Standard Score; IQ*; and *percentage of schooling spent in special school*. Finally, the genetic groups, deletion and disomy, were compared on mean underachievement scores.

The correlates of underachievement clearly differed for the PWS and LD groups. For the LD group, no variable significantly affected underachievement across the academic domains, but for the PWS group, both *Vineland Socialisation Domain Standard Score* and *percentage of schooling in special school* correlated significantly with underachievement across all three academic domains. For both groups, *underachievement in arithmetic* correlated with *age* and *underachievement in reading* correlated with *BMI*.[20] Using multiple regression analysis, for the LD group there was no significant predictor of underachievement, but for the PWS group *percentage of schooling spent in special school* remained a significant predictor for all three academic domains.[20]

Strikingly, among people with PWS, mean underachievement varied by academic domain and by genetic subgroup (see Figure 7.8). Differences in mean underachievement between those with deletion and those with disomy were greatest in reading, slightly smaller in spelling and very small in arithmetic. The disomy subgroup actually reached the expected attainment level in reading. The differences in degree of underachievement between the subgroups in reading and spelling were approximately half of the standard deviations within subgroups.

The genotype common to all people with PWS clearly has a major effect on the cognitive phenotype and resultant attainments, but there are interesting differences

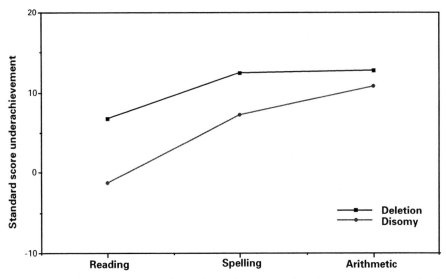

Figure 7.8.   Mean underachievement of Prader–Willi syndrome genetic subgroups across academic domains.

between genetic subtypes and, most importantly, evidence that the nature of the education received affects outcome for people with this syndrome.

The finding that the percentage of time in schooling spent in special needs schools is a significant predictor of underachievement in the PWS group, but not in the LD group, is not easily explained. Anecdotally we know that some children with PWS are placed in special needs schools, not because of low IQ, but because of behavioural problems (e.g. temper tantrums and stealing food or money to buy food), which are not routinely dealt with in mainstream school. Correlations between *aberrant behaviour* and *percentage time in special needs schools* were 0.21 (children) and 0.25 (adults) in the PWS group and 0.01 and −0.08 in the LD group, which gives some support to the anecdotal evidence. However, this cannot be the whole explanation because correlations between underachievement and behavioural measures were not significant.[20] Further investigation also revealed that IQ differences did not account for time in special needs school in either group (see Table 7.5). Significantly, all seven people (five PWS, two LD) who were achieving at expected levels in all three academic domains had never, or had not yet, been to a special needs school, while of 19 (11 PWS, eight LD) with IQ > 40 who were below the cut-off points on all three attainment tests, only three had less than 100% schooling in special needs schools (one in the LD group 55%; one with PWS transferred at age five years; one in the PWS group with a psychiatric illness whose attainment levels had clearly been higher in the past). On the other hand, as shown in Table 7.5, some people who had spent more than half their schooling in special needs schools were achieving at expected levels in at least one academic domain. This seems to indicate that it is not

Table 7.5. Percentage of schooling in special needs schools and IQ and numbers at various levels of achievement

	Percentage of schooling in special needs schools		
	0	1–50	51–100
PWS group (n = 71)			
Number	21 (30%)	8 (11%)	42 (59%)
Mean IQ ($\geq$40)	73	66.5	62
IQ range	51–103	49–84	46–82 (3 $\leq$ 40)[a]
Read. $\geq$ expect	13	3	8
Spell. $\geq$ expect	10	2	2
Arith. $\geq$ expect	9	0	1
All $\geq$ expect	5	0	0
Read. < cut-off	0	0	13
Spell. < cut-off	0	0	12
Arith. < cut-off	0	0	15
All < cut-off	0	0	11
LD group (n = 40)			
Number	9 (22.5%)	6 (15%)	25 (62.5%)
Mean IQ ($\geq$40)	82	75	60.5
IQ range	65–99	53–86	41–86 (4 $\leq$ 40)[a]
Read. $\geq$ expect	4	1	2
Spell. $\geq$ expect	3	0	1
Arith. $\geq$ expect	2	1	0
All $\geq$ expect	2	0	0
Read. < cut-off	0	0	9
Spell. < cut-off	1	0	8
Arith. < cut-off	0	0	11
All < cut-off	0	0	8

[a] Omitted from IQ means and ranges and achievement numbers.

PWS: Prader–Willi syndrome; LD: learning disabilities.

the type of school per se that fosters underachievement, but that some special needs schools are less likely than mainstream schools to teach basic reading, spelling and arithmetic to children who are difficult to accommodate. This may be because their general ability levels are higher than those of their classmates, or appear lower than they really are because of immature behaviour, or because of expectations based on their school placement. Of the basic skills, reading is the most likely to be tackled in a special needs school and is 'a strength of people with PWS', which might explain the number of those in the PWS group, 51–100% of whose schooling had been in special needs schools, who do achieve expected levels in reading.

Underachievement patterns were different for the PWS and LD groups. The PWS group was better at reading than arithmetic, with spelling intermediate, whereas the LD group were equally good at reading and arithmetic and worse at spelling. The PWS group had lower levels of underachievement in reading and spelling than the LD group but performance in arithmetic was similar. It seems that, relative to other people with LD, people with PWS have relative strengths in reading and spelling, but not in arithmetic.

In both the PWS and the LD groups, underachievement in arithmetic was significantly correlated with IQ. This may indicate that the regression equations derived from the normalisation samples for the Wechsler and WRAT attainment tests break down for the arithmetic test at lower levels of IQ. However, the lack of significant correlations with IQ for underachievement in reading and spelling suggests that the regression equations for these do hold at lower IQ levels. We are unable to offer any explanation of the correlation between underachievement in reading and BMI in both PWS and LD groups. The level of significance is not large (0.05), so this may just be a consequence of the number of significance tests conducted.

As the scatter plots show, underachievement is not universal in either the PWS or the LD groups, but the average attainments are below the predicted levels. Through correlation analysis two systematic influences on underachievement have been identified for the PWS group: school type, as discussed above; and Vineland Socialisation Domain Standard Score. The latter may be interpreted as a proxy for some of the factors hypothesised to be instrumental in achievement in normal children via their influence on the ability to interact with others; for example, motivation, response to encouragement, pleasing others and competing. We also formed the view that certain other factors may have affected the attainment levels of particular individuals but without any systematic effect in either PWS or LD groups. These factors included gender, number of siblings (divided attention from their parents, competition), BMI and severity of eating disorder (intrusive thoughts of food or body image), daytime sleepiness, aberrant behaviour, and attention deficit, hyperactivity and autistic traits. We were not able to include some possibly relevant variables such as teaching methods. We suspect that teaching based on concrete materials, rule-based learning and visual methods would be better for people with PWS, who have poor auditory short-term memory, difficulty in generalising and do not understand abstract concepts.

Finally, we found that the patterns of underachievement across academic domains differ for deletion and disomy genetic subgroups of people with PWS. On average, the disomy subgroup showed no underachievement in reading. The greater underachievement in the deletion group may be explained by the greater average percentage of schooling spent in special schools or by the lower VIQ compared with PIQ means of the deletion group relative to the disomy group.

In the UK it is the process of 'statementing' that is the gateway to receiving special educational help. This process may need to consider the cause of a person's disability and its impact on cognitive, social and emotional development if it is to ensure that all people with LD receive the form of education that results in the best possible outcomes. Whilst the cognitive development of people with specific genetic disorders may be constrained by the effect on brain development, levels of attainment may well be significantly altered depending on the individual's educational environment.

REFERENCES

1. Sulzbacher, S. J., Crnic, K. A. & Snow, J. Behavioral and cognitive disabilities in Prader–Willi syndrome. In Holm, V. A., Sulzbacher, S. J. & Pipes, P. L. (Eds). *The Prader–Willi Syndrome*. Baltimore: University Park Press, 1981.

2. Falconer, D. S. *Introduction to Quantitative Genetics*. New York: Longman, 1981.

3. Curfs, L. M. G., Wiegers, A. M., Sommers, J. R. M., Borghgraef, M. & Fryns, J. P. Strengths and weaknesses in the cognitive profile of youngsters with Prader–Willi syndrome. *Clinical Genetics* **40** (1991), 430–434.

4. Curfs, L. M. G. & Fryns, J.-P. Prader–Willi syndrome: a review with special attention to the cognitive and behavioral profile. *Birth Defects: Original Article Series* **28** (1992), 99–104.

5. Holm, V. A. Medical management of Prader–Willi syndrome. In Holm, V. A., Sulzbacher, S. J. & Pipes, P. L. (Eds). *The Prader–Willi Syndrome*. Baltimore: University Park Press, 1981.

6. Dykens, E. M., Hodapp, R. M., Walsh, K. & Nash, L. J. Profiles, correlates, and trajectories of intelligence in Prader–Willi syndrome. *American Academy of Child and Adolescent Psychiatry* **31** (1992), 1125–1129.

7. Warren, H. L. & Hunt, E. Cognitive processing in children with Prader–Willi syndrome. In Holm, V. A., Sulzbacher, S. J. & Pipes, P. L. (Eds). *The Prader–Willi Syndrome*. Baltimore: University Park Press, 1981.

8. Cassidy, S. B. Prader–Willi syndrome. *Journal of Medical Genetics* **34** (1997), 917–923.

9. Roof, E., Stone, W., MacLean, W., Feurer, I. D., Thompson, T. & Butler, M. G. Intellectual characteristics of Prader–Willi syndrome: comparison of genetic subtypes. *Journal of Intellectual Disability Research* **44** (2000), 25–30.

10. Dykens, E. M. Are jigsaw puzzle skills 'spared' in people with Prader–Willi syndrome? *Journal of Child Psychology and Psychiatry* **43** (2002), 343–352.

11. Wechsler, D. *The Wechsler Adult Intelligence Scale (WAIS-Revised UK Edition), Wechsler Intelligence Scale for Children (WISC lll –UK), Pre-school and Primary Scale of Intelligence (WPPSI-Revised UK)*. Psychological Corporation. London: Harcourt Brace & Co, 1993.

12. Whittington, J. E., Holland, A. J., Webb, T., Butler, J. V., Clarke, D. J. & Boer, H. Cognitive abilities and genotype in a population-based sample of people with Prader–Willi syndrome. *Journal of Intellectual Disability Research* **48** (2003), 172–187.

13. Malich, S., Largo, R. H., Schinzel, A., Molinari, L. & Eiholzer, U. Phenotypic heterogeneity of growth and psychometric intelligence in Prader–Willi syndrome: variable expression of a contiguous gene syndrome or parent-child resemblance? *American Journal of Medical Genetics* **91** (2000), 298–304.

14. Hashimoto, T., Mori, K., Yoneda, Y. *et al.* Proton magnetic spectroscopy of the brain in patients with Prader–Willi syndrome. *Pediatric Neurology* **18** (1998), 30–35.

15. Cassidy, S. B., Forsythe, M., Heeger, S. *et al.* Comparison of phenotype between patients with Prader–Willi syndrome due to deletion 15q and uniparental disomy 15. *American Journal of Medical Genetics* **68** (1997), 433–440.

16. Dykens, E. M. Psychopathology in children with intellectual disability. *Journal of Child Psychology and Psychiatry* **41** (2000), 407–417.

17. Rust, J. *Wechsler Objective Language Dimensions (WOLD), Wechsler Objective Numerical Dimensions (WOND)*. Psychological Corporation. London: Harcourt Brace & Co, 1995.

18. Wechsler, D. *Wechsler Objective Reading Dimensions (WORD)*. London: Psychological Corporation. Harcourt Brace & Co, 1993.

19. Wilkinson, G. S. *The Wide Range Achievement Test (WRAT-3)* London: Psychological Corporation. Harcourt Brace & Co, 1993.

20. Whittington, J. E., Holland, A. J., Webb, T., Butler, J. V., Clarke, D. J. & Boer H. Under-achievement in Prader–Willi Syndrome. *Journal of Intellectual Disability Research* **48** (2003), 188–200.

8

The behavioural phenotype of PWS

The concept of 'behavioural phenotypes in organic genetic diseases' was first proposed by Nyhan in his Presidential lecture to the American Paediatric Association in 1971.[1] He was referring to the fact that severe self-injurious behaviour was as much a part of the phenotype of the X-linked syndrome that subsequently was named the Lesch–Nyhan syndrome, as was any physical abnormality. In the last few years the association between specific genetically determined developmental syndromes and particular cognitive, linguistic and behavioural profiles has been increasingly recognised.[2,3,4,5] This has partly been due to advances in genetic techniques, particularly in the identification of novel genetic mechanisms that give rise to developmental disorders and can account for phenotypic variation within syndromes. The best example of the latter is the relevance of the CGG triplet repeat sequence length in people with Fragile X syndrome.[6]

In the case of genetic syndromes associated with a 'behavioural phenotype', it is proposed that single genes may have specific effects on brain development and function, and thereby give rise to particular patterns of social, emotional and/or cognitive development, and an increased propensity to aberrant behaviours that are recognised as being specifically, but not exclusively, associated with that syndrome.[7] This association between genetic syndromes and 'behavioural phenotypes' is in contrast to the usual model of behavioural 'normality', which presumes an interaction between the inheritance of allelic variants of several genes and shared or non-shared environmental influences on cognitive development, and on behaviour patterns and personality.[8]

The evidence for behavioural phenotypes in organic genetic disorders has been mainly based on statistical associations. People with a genetic abnormality have characteristic behaviour patterns that are atypical among the rest of the population, and different genetic abnormalities are associated with different sets of characteristic behaviours.[9] A more direct link can be established by genetic 'knock-out' animal models, in which animals are bred with a target genetic defect and the resultant aberrant behaviour observed. For example, knock-out of the imprinted gene *mest* in mice is associated with abnormal maternal behaviour and growth retardation.[10]

Flint & Yule[2] have proposed stringent criteria that need to be met before a syndrome can be said to have a 'behavioural phenotype', and stated that they were aware of only three syndromes meeting these criteria: Lesch–Nyhan, Prader–Willi, and Rett syndromes. In these syndromes the genetic defects are, respectively, a mutation in a single gene on the X chromosome (Xq26–27), an abnormality of expression of maternally imprinted genes located on the proximal long arm of chromosome 15 (15q11–13), and a dominant mutation of the *MECP2* gene on the X chromosome, which is incompatible with viable male fetal development. The outstanding associated aberrant behaviours are, respectively, self-injurious behaviour, excessive interest in food and severe over-eating in the absence of restriction of access to food, and a severe progressive neurological disorder with fits of screaming or laughter and stereotyped hand movements. Using the broad definition of 'behavioural phenotype' that includes cognitive, linguistic and/or behavioural profiles, other syndromes may also be included, for example, Williams syndrome with its specific pattern of language development,[11,12] or syndromes not necessarily associated with significant learning disabilities, such as myotonic dystrophy, where severe apathy is a characteristic feature.[13]

Questionnaire-based studies using the Aberrant Behaviour Checklist have shown that people with PWS have a characteristic behaviour profile in which temper outbursts (including aggressive behaviour and screaming), self harm (especially skin picking), mood swings and repetitive speech are common.[14] In addition, repetitive questioning, compulsive behaviours and hoarding are more common and it has been proposed that an obsessive–compulsive disorder is frequently present,[15] although this has been disputed and reinterpreted as a specific developmental delay.[16] The most striking behaviour is that of severe and persistent over-eating, which, if unrestricted, leads to life-threatening obesity. Increasingly now, this behaviour, although still potentially present, is unreported because a better knowledge of the syndrome has led to tight restrictions over access to food and therefore the behaviour of over-eating cannot occur. It has been proposed that the propensity to this behaviour is due to a failure of the normal feedback mechanisms that lead to a state of satiation following food intake.[17] With respect to adaptive behaviours, as measured by the Vineland Adaptive Behaviour Scales, there are strengths in the Daily Living Skills domain, and weaknesses in the Socialisation domain.[18]

The genotype of PWS has been described in Chapters 1 and 5. Both imprinted and non-imprinted genes contribute to the physical phenotype and the same is probably true of the behavioural phenotype. The evidence for the contribution of imprinted genes is summarised in Chapter 5. For example, it is thought that the characteristic 'fair hair and skin compared to family background' included in the consensus diagnostic criteria, which is found in varying proportions of people with PWS, is due to the loss of one copy of a non-imprinted pigmentation gene. In the case of a full deletion of the PWS region, or of maternal isodisomy, only one copy or two identical copies, respectively, of this gene will be available and so the chances of inheriting the recessive fair colouring will be increased. Comparisons between those with the deletion form, and those with chromosome 15 heterodisomies are one means of trying to separate out the effects of maternally imprinted genes by themselves (i.e. those with disomies), from the effects of maternally imprinted genes and the loss of a single copy of other non-imprinted genes at that chromosomal locus. Relatively few differences have so far been found (see Chapter 6): disomy is tentatively associated with higher average maternal age, less 'fair for family' colouring (as above), higher average verbal ability and less severe eating and other problems.[19] More recently, it has been found that severe psychiatric illness is more common in people with chromosome 15 maternal disomies, and may in fact be inevitable in early adult life. The same is not true for those with deletion and it has been proposed that a maternally or paternally imprinted gene on chromosome 15, and the resultant gene dosage effect, may be a cause of psychotic illness in the general population.[20]

Whilst the concept of 'behavioural phenotypes' in general is now receiving increasing attention, there has been a limited focus on the potential underlying brain mechanisms that might mediate between genes and behaviour in genetic syndromes. Hodapp,[7] in a conceptual paper, considered possible direct and indirect (environmental) effects. He argued that in individual syndromes, characteristic physical and behavioural features were not invariably present (referred to as 'consistency'), and went on to propose that behavioural phenotypes were therefore best conceptualised as 'the heightened probability' that such behaviour will occur in a given syndrome. He gives considerable weight to the potential influence of environmental interactions on the shaping of specific behaviours, and thereby to their increased occurrence in those with the syndrome. Dykens et al.[19] proposed that some of the obsessive behaviours – skin picking and nail-biting – may be a form of excessive grooming. They argued that this might in turn reflect abnormalities of oxytocin and/or 5-HT function in the hypothalamus. Ultimately such models must be able to account for the full range and combinations of behaviours that affect people with PWS, the observations that such behaviours are not necessarily invariable, and for any changes in behaviour profile observed across the lifespan.

We have chosen to take a more reductionist approach, and have recently proposed possible developmental and neurobiological mechanisms that might account for how genes impact on behaviour in those with genetic syndromes.[21] The benefits of such conceptual models are, first, they enable testable hypotheses to be developed for both PWS and other syndromes with 'behavioural phenotypes' and, second, they provide a means for considering possible 'actions' for the products of the specific gene(s) associated with that syndrome. Such models will not explain the minutiae or variations in the intensity of the associated behaviours, and should certainly not be taken to imply that such behaviours are unchangeable, but may account for the increased propensity to the behaviour among those with the syndrome. We strongly argue that such an approach has the potential for significant therapeutic benefits. The general models proposed include the following:

- *All or none model.* The impaired expression of a single gene has a direct effect on the behavioural characteristic(s). We would hypothesise that in the case of a probable contiguous gene syndrome, such as PWS, the protein product of one of a number of genes making up the genotype would be found to have an action, and a site of expression, that directly influences the behaviour. In this case the effect is always present when the gene is not expressed, and we predict that this aspect of the phenotype would be close to being universal across the syndrome, and independent of other behaviours.

- *Threshold shift model.* The effect of a gene is to shift the mean of a normal population distribution of a behaviour towards one extreme, thus increasing the proportion above a particular threshold and therefore the likelihood of it being seen as abnormal. This liability threshold model is similar to that proposed in the general population to explain the increased liability to specific psychiatric disorders in those with a family history of that disorder. Thus, for those with the specific genetic syndrome, there should be a correlation between the 'index behaviour' and associated traits in first degree relatives.

- *Arrested development model.* The effect of a gene is to interfere with normal brain development so that it is arrested or severely delayed or deviant.[7,22] With this model, the behaviour in question will be characteristic of that normally found transiently at a younger age, will persist across ages, and there will be evidence of developmental arrest in those with the syndrome at an age when this behaviour normally occurs.

The Cambridge study investigated the profile of adaptive behaviour, and the nature and extent of specific behaviours in an augmented population-based sample of both children and adults with PWS. In addition, we investigated the relationship of specific behaviours to each other, as well as to other variables such as age and Body Mass Index (BMI). In order to look at the clustering of behavioural characteristics in PWS, we carried out a factor analysis. Here we report on: (1) the behavioural differences between people with PWS and those with learning disabilities (LD) of other aetiologies, and on the prevalence of these behaviours; and (2) putative mechanisms to explain differences in the prevalence rates of specific behaviours, and explore how far our data support one or more of the models described earlier to account for these findings.

The methodology for the collection of the data and the instruments used are described in Chapter 3. Participants in the research described in this chapter included 65 people with PWS, identified as part of the population-based study, who volunteered for participation in the main phenotypic study, together with 26 volunteers with PWS from other areas of the UK and a comparison group of 42 people with LD not due to PWS. Mean age of the PWS group was 20.8 years and that of the comparison group was 20.2 years; mean IQ of the PWS group was 62.9 and that of the comparison group was 64.1.

The instruments relevant to what is reported in this Chapter included those sections of the PWS Questionnaire (Chapter 3, Appendix 3.1), which contain behavioural aspects of the diagnostic criteria. The behaviours rated were: *eating behaviour; skin picking; temper tantrums; repetitive questions; obsessive behaviour; violent or aggressive outbursts; mood swings; argumentativeness; stealing; lying, stubbornness;* and (from the Vineland scales) *possessiveness*. Most behaviours were rated on a scale of 0 to 4 taking into account both severity and frequency. The exceptions were '*stubborn*' and '*possessive*' which occurred in different parts of the interview and were rated on a 3-point scale. In addition, the following established informant interviews were used: the Developmental Behaviour Checklist[23] for children (up to and including those aged 17) and the Aberrant Behaviour Checklist[24] for adults. Both these instruments have been used to determine the range of behaviours associated with specific syndromes, and published data are available. For both children and adults intellectual ability was established using the relevant Wechsler Scales,[25] and Adaptive Behaviours were assessed using the full version of the Vineland Adaptive Behaviour Scales.[26]

Analysis of the data indicated that there were no significant differences in behavioural profile between the population-based cohort and those living outside the Anglia & Oxford Health Region. Prevalence rates are reported for the population-based cohort but the cohorts are combined when relationships between particular aspects of the phenotype are examined.

The prevalence rates of PWS physical and behavioural 'diagnostic' signs and symptoms and their severity are shown in Tables 8.1 and 8.2. Table 8.1 clearly shows the existence of characteristics present in a high proportion of people with PWS (73–98% definitely affected) and other less prevalent characteristics. For the comparison group, there is also a range of prevalence rates, but only prevalence of the matching characteristic (learning disability) is comparable with the highest rates found in the PWS group. All the criteria in Table 8.1 were significantly more prevalent (chi-square $P < 0.001$) in the PWS group, *fair for family* ($P < 0.01$) and *articulation difficulties* ($P < 0.05$) were also more prevalent, but the differences were less significant. Similarly, all the behaviours in Table 8.2 were significantly more prevalent ($P < 0.001$) in the PWS group, except that *possessiveness* was not as

Table 8.1. Prader–Willi syndrome (PWS) criteria in population sample

Criterion	%Definite		%Mild		%None	
	PWS	LD	PWS	LD	PWS	LD
Floppy at birth	98	24	2	6	0	70
Poor suck	97	21	3	0	0	79
Feeding difficulties	97	46	3	3	0	51
Decreased movement during pregnancy	68	14	5	7	27	79
Weak cry/inactivity	94	15	6	12	0	73
Obesity/rapid weight gain	79	50	2	6	19	44
Food obsession/overeat	78	57	5	13	17	30
Abnormal/delayed sexual – males	98	23	2	6	0	71
– females	73	31	27	8	0	62
Learning disabilities	94	95	6	3	0	3
Short height <10th centile	81	42	2	0	17	58
Small hands or feet	85	27	11	21	3	52
Fair for family	6	8	50	33	44	58
Reported scoliosis	26	3	8	11	66	86
Eye problems	78	54	3	0	19	46
Thick/excessive saliva	51	0	16	3	32 + 2	97
Articulation difficulties	68	58	18	15	15	27
Sleep disturbance	60	43	8	5	30 + 2	51
High pain threshold	56	10	30	43	14	47
Sensitivity hot/cold	44	14	22	0	33	86
Jigsaws	38	0	16	8	46	92
Decreased vomiting	41	11	41	23	19	66

LD: learning disabilities.

strongly significant ($P < 0.05$), and *argumentative* and *lying* were not significantly different between the two groups.

Turning to maladaptive behaviour, Table 8.3 gives details of full-scale and sub-scale scores for children with PWS and a comparison group with non-specific LD. None of the comparisons reached statistical significance. There was a tendency for the PWS group to score higher on the *Communication Disturbance* and *Autistic Traits* scales and lower on the other four scales. In both groups, average scores exceeded 1 on four items: *distractible; temper tantrums; no sense of danger;* and *stubborn*. Average scores exceeded 1 in the PWS group on a further eight behaviour items relating to obsessiveness (*ordering, obsessive, repetitive speech, routine*), poor peer relationships (*prefers company of older or younger people, loner*), skin picking and *overall problem severity*, the latter being only slightly lower in the LD group.

Table 8.2. Prader–Willi syndrome (PWS) behaviours in population sample

Criterion	%Definite	%Mild	%None
Eating behaviour – PWS	76	22	2
– LD	*41*	*21*	*38*
Skin picking – PWS	55	23	22
– LD	*11*	*24*	*65*
Temper tantrums – PWS	66	31	3
– LD	*50*	*21*	*29*
Violence – PWS	41	32	27
– LD	*36*	*14*	*50*
Mood fluctuations – PWS	38	19	44
– LD	*22*	*20*	*58*
Repetitive questions – PWS	66	11	23
– LD	*24*	*21*	*55*
Obsessional traits – PWS	69	22	9
– LD	*25*	*47*	*28*
Argumentative – PWS	37	25	37
– LD	*34*	*19*	*47*
Lying – PWS	28	26	46
– LD	*27*	*30*	*43*
Stealing – PWS	42	28	30
– LD	*23*	*11*	*66*
Stubborn – PWS	85	10	3 + 2
– LD	*60*	*16*	*24*
Possessive – PWS	55	23	23
– LD	*44*	*19*	*36*

LD: learning disabilities.

Average scores exceeded 1 in the LD group on a further four behaviour items: *poor attention span; cries easily; easily led;* and *impatient*. The first and last of these being only slightly lower in the PWS group.

Maladaptive behaviour in adults was measured by the Aberrant Behaviour Checklist. Behavioural profiles are shown in Table 8.4 as full-scale and sub-scale scores. Average scores were higher in the PWS group, compared with the LD group, on all scales, and reached statistical significance (*t*-test, $P < 0.01$) for the *full-scale score* and the *irritability scale*. Table 8.4 also shows that the number of serious/severe ratings was higher in the PWS group. In the PWS group, two items had average scores greater than 1 (*temper tantrums* and *demands must be met immediately*) and a further five items had average scores of 0.9 or higher (*inactive, repetitive speech,*

Table 8.3. Aberrant behaviours in full Prader–Willi syndrome (PWS) sample – children

Variable	Group	Mean	Std Dev.	Min.	Max.	*n*
DBC total score	PWS	**44.7**	**22.1**	**9**	93	33
	LD	46.7	27.6	8	94	19
Disruptive scale	PWS	**11.8**	**7.5**	**0**	32	33
	LD	14.8	10.5	2	35	19
Self-absorbed scale	PWS	**7.2**	**5.1**	**1**	21	33
	LD	9.4	6.7	0	21	19
Communication	PWS	**4.7**	**2.7**	**0**	11	33
	LD	3.3	2.8	0	9	19
Anxiety scale	PWS	**5.6**	**3.5**	**0**	16	33
	LD	6.4	4.0	0	13	19
Autistic trait scale	PWS	**3.7**	**3.5**	**0**	11	33
	LD	2.4	2.0	0	6	19
Antisocial scale	PWS	**1.7**	**2.0**	**0**	6	33
	LD	2.0	2.3	0	8	19

Number of individual items with average score > 1:
> In PWS group 12 items (ordering, distractible, obsessive, temper tantrums, no sense danger, company old or younger, loner, repetitive speech, skin picks, stubborn, routine, problems).
> In learning disabilities (LD) group 8 items (attention span, cries easily, distractible, easily led, temper tantrums, impatient, no sense danger, stubborn).

Number of individual items with average score ≥0.9:
> In PWS group 5 items (aloof, attention, impatient, talks too much, high pain).
> In LD group 1 item (problems).

DBC: Development Behaviour Checklist; Std Dev: standard deviation.

not attending to instructions, distractible, and *tantrums if doesn't get own way).* In the LD group, the highest average item score was 0.8 for the item: *difficult to reach.* The comparison between Tables 8.3 and 8.4 is cross-sectional and the straightforward interpretation that people with non-specific LDs may grow out of the aberrant behaviours, but people with PWS do not, may be too simplistic (see discussion below).

Adaptive behaviour was measured by the Vineland Adaptive Behaviour Scales. Tables 8.5 and 8.6 show the domain standard scores and the sub-domain age eqi-valents of the PWS and LD groups for children and adults. There are no significant differences between group means (*t*-test) in any of the domain standard scores or sub-domain age equivalents, but on the *maladaptive behaviour scale* adult means are significantly higher in the PWS group (*P* < 0.01). Relative to the LD group, the PWS adult group show a weakness on the *coping skills sub-domain* and a strength

Table 8.4. Aberrant behaviours in full Prader–Willi syndrome (PWS) sample – adults

Variable	Group	Mean	Std Dev.	Min.	Max.	n
ABC Total score	PWS	**28.6**** **(2.3)**	**20.2 (3.7)**	**1 (0)**	82 (18)	50
	LD	17.1 (0.8)	13.1 (1.0)	2 (0)	46 (3)	15
Irritability scale	PWS	**9.4**** **(0.9)**	**7.5 (1.6)**	**0 (0)**	27 (6)	50
	LD	4.6 (0.3)	5.6 (0.8)	0 (0)	16 (3)	15
Lethargy scale	PWS	**7.8 (0.6)**	**7.3 (1.2)**	**0 (0)**	28 (6)	50
	LD	4.6 (0.2)	6.9 (0.4)	0 (0)	26 (1)	15
Stereotypy scale	PWS	**1.9 (0.2)**	**3.0 (0.6)**	**0 (0)**	12 (3)	50
	LD	1.7 (0)	2.7 (0)	0 (0)	8 (0)	15
Hyperactivity scale	PWS	**6.9 (0.4)**	**5.6 (1.0)**	**0 (0)**	22 (5)	50
	LD	4.5 (0.1)	5.0 (0.4)	0 (0)	16 (0)	15
Inappropriate speech	PWS	**2.7 (0.3)**	**2.9 (0.8)**	**0 (0)**	11 (3)	50
	LD	1.7 (0.1)	2.3 (0.4)	0 (0)	7 (1)	15

**Significant $P < 0.01$.

Figures in parentheses refer to numbers of serious/severe rating scores

Number of individual items with average score > 1:

In PWS group 2 items (temper tantrums, demands must be met immediately).

In learning disabilities (LD) group 0 items.

Number of individual items with average score ≥ 0.9:

In PWS group 5 items (inactive, repetitive speech, not attend instructions, distractible, own way or tantrums).

In LD group 0 items (highest average. 8, difficult to reach).

ABC: Aberrant Behaviour Checklist; Std Dev: standard deviation.

on the *Community sub-domain*. This is also reflected in the standard scores (all ages combined) on the three domains, shown in Figure 8.1, where people with PWS have relative strengths in *daily living skills* and relative weaknesses in *socialisation skills*.

In order to test some of the hypotheses we have proposed that would account for the manifestation of specific aspects of the PWS behavioural phenotype, we have assessed the relationships between specific variables, and between these and various behaviours. The effects of *age, IQ, severity of eating disorder* and *current BMI* were investigated by correlation analysis, among themselves, then with the diagnostic criteria, the behavioural criteria, the maladaptive behaviour checklists, and finally, with Vineland scores. We reported the many correlations investigated, but specifically examined those that enabled our hypotheses to be tested. We have retained the 0.05 significance level, and the significance levels are indicated as * $= 0.05$, ** $= 0.01$, *** $= 0.001$ with the significant findings reported.

Table 8.5. Adaptive behaviours – children

Domain/Sub-domain	Group	Mean	S.D.	Min.	Max.	n
Communication age equivalents						
Receptive	PWS	3.6	1.7	0.5	7.8	37
	LD	3.7	1.9	0.9	7.8	17
Expressive	PWS	3.6	1.9	0.5	7.4	37
	LD	4.4	2.2	1.0	8.8	17
Written	PWS	5.3	2.9	1.3	11.8	37
	LD	6.6	2.1	1.3	8.8	17
Daily Living Skills age equivalents						
Personal	PWS	3.6	1.8	0.7	8.3	37
	LD	4.6	2.6	0.7	10.2	17
Domestic	PWS	4.0	2.2	1.3	8.9	37
	LD	4.6	3.0	1.3	12.3	17
Community	PWS	4.2	2.6	0.4	9.3	37
	LD	5.2	2.7	0.4	9.5	17
Socialisation age equivalents						
Interpersonal	PWS	3.4	1.9	0.4	7.8	37
	LD	5.0	4.1	0.6	15.0	17
Play & leisure	PWS	3.3	2.1	0.5	9.7	37
	LD	4.1	3.0	1.3	13.3	17
Coping skills	PWS	3.3	1.6	0.8	6.1	37
	LD	3.7	2.3	0.8	8.9	17
Motor Skills age equivalents						
Gross motor	PWS	2.3	1.3	0.3	5.3	35
	LD	3.0	1.6	0.7	5.9	10
Fine motor	PWS	3.3	1.8	0.1	5.1	35
	LD	3.4	1.7	0.1	5.1	10
Communication standard	PWS	58	17	27	92	37
	LD	56	18	38	110	17
Daily Living standard	PWS	50	20	20	95	37
	LD	44	16	20	71	17
Socialisation standard	PWS	59	15	27	89	37
	LD	56	8	45	76	17
Maladaptive behaviour scores I	PWS	1.24	0.74	0	2	29
	LD	1.20	0.91	0	2	16

PWS: Prader–Willi syndrome; LD: learning disabilities.

Table 8.6. Adaptive behaviours – adults

Domain/Sub-domain	Group	Mean	S.D.	Min.	Max.	n
Communication age equivalents						
Receptive	PWS	5.0	1.7	1.8	7.8	43
	LD	3.9	0.9	2.1	4.8	13
Expressive	PWS	6.0	2.7	1.8	15.5	42
	LD	4.9	2.5	0.9	8.8	12
Written	PWS	8.7	4.1	1.3	18.8	42
	LD	6.5	3.2	1.3	10.3	12
Daily Living Skills age equivalents						
Personal	PWS	7.1	3.3	2.3	17.5	43
	LD	6.3	2.2	1.5	8.7	12
Domestic	PWS	8.1	3.6	2.5	18.9	43
	LD	7.3	3.2	1.9	11.8	13
Community	PWS	7.7	3.4	2.2	16.3	41
	LD	6.4	2.8	1.0	10.0	13
Socialisation age equivalents						
Interpersonal	PWS	6.5	3.0	2.0	14.8	41
	LD	5.3	2.8	0.1	8.7	12
Play & leisure	PWS	5.9	3.2	2.0	15.8	41
	LD	5.2	3.1	1.2	9.5	11
Coping skills	PWS	5.4	2.0	2.0	11.3	42
	LD	5.6	2.2	1.4	8.9	13
Motor Skills age equivalents						
Gross motor	PWS	2.5	1.3	0.8	5.9	24
	LD	3.1	1.9	1.8	5.9	4
Fine motor	PWS	4.7	0.9	2.0	5.1	23
	LD	2.8	1.3	1.1	4.1	4
Communication standard	PWS	40	21	20	97	40
	LD	31	10	20	46	12
Daily Living standard	PWS	43	19	20	80	40
	LD	39	17	20	62	12
Socialisation standard	PWS	39	14	20	68	41
	LD	37	13	20	51	11
Maladaptive behaviour scores I	PWS	1.02	0.61	0	2	46
	LD	0.38	0.51	0	1	13
Maladaptive behaviour scores II	PWS	0.83	0.57	0	2	35
	LD	0.31	0.48	0	1	13

PWS: Prader–Willi syndrome; LD: learning disabilities.

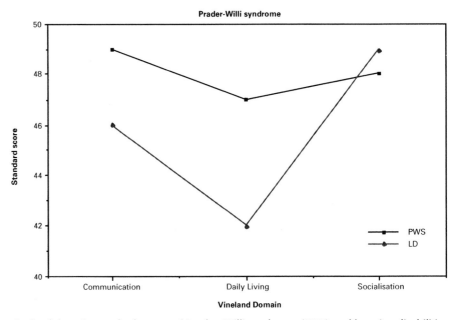

Figure 8.1.   Vineland domain standard scores of Prader–Willi syndrome (PWS) and learning disabilities (LD) groups – all ages.

There were three significant correlations between *age, severity of eating disorder* and *current BMI* in the PWS group, but only one in the LD group. In both groups, *age* and *BMI* were positively correlated (**PWS; ***LD), and in the PWS group, *severity of eating disorder* correlated positively with both *age*** and *BMI*. The correlation between *BMI* and *age* in the PWS reflected the fact that management guidelines were not available and diagnosis had often been made at a greater age in the older PWS population, and access to food had not been controlled. Also, certain characteristics (e.g. stature) and behaviours (e.g. lying and stealing) become more noticeable, more inappropriate, and/or more difficult to manage with age. Tables 8.7 to 8.9 show all the significant correlations between *age, severity of eating disorder, current BMI* and diagnostic criteria and characteristic behaviours (Table 8.7), and behaviour checklists, aberrant behaviour, and Vineland scales (Tables 8.8 and 8.9).

The absence of correlations between IQ and diagnostic criteria in the PWS group distinguished them from the LD group, where the presence of these clinical characteristics correlates with lower IQ. In children, behavioural criteria and IQ were uncorrelated for both groups, but for adults with PWS, more severe problematic behaviour correlated with lower IQ. The Vineland domain standard scores are adjusted for age, so that the negative correlations imply increasing developmental

Table 8.7. Correlates of age, IQ, severity of eating disorder and current Body Mass Index (BMI) with diagnostic criteria and behaviour characteristics

		PWS	LD		PWS	LD
Age	Childhood obesity	+ ***		Violence/aggression	− *	
	Overeat/food obsession	+ ***		Temper tantrums		− *
	Short height	+ *		Argumentativeness		− *
	Small hands/feet	+ ***		Lying	+ *	
	Eye problems	+ **		Stealing	+ ***	
	High pain threshold	+ **		Possessiveness		+ ***
	Temperature irregularities	+ **		Stubbornness		− **
	Articulation	− ***	+ *			
IQ	Floppiness at birth		− **	Temper tantrums	− **	
	Learning difficulties	− ***		Violence/aggression	− **	
	Childhood obesity		− **	Mood swings	− **	
	Periods/year (females)		+ *	Repetitive questions	− *	
	Short height		− *	Lying	+ **	
	Articulation		− ***	Stealing		+ *
	Skill with jigsaws	+ *		Possessiveness	− *	
Eating	Childhood obesity	+ ***		Skin picking	+ **	
	Overeat/food obsession	+ ***	+ ***	Temper tantrums		+ ***
	Disturbed/noisy sleep		+ *	Repetitive questions	+ ***	+ **
	Eye problems	+ **		Obsessiveness	+ **	+ ***
	High pain threshold	+ ***		Argumentativeness		+ *
	Temperature irregularities	+ ***		Lying	+ ***	+ ***
	Skill with jigsaws		− *	Stealing	+ ***	+ ***
				Possessiveness		+ *
BMI	Floppiness at birth		− *	Obsessiveness	− *	
	Childhood obesity	+ ***	+ ***	Possessiveness		− *
	Overeat/food obsession	+ **				
	Periods/year (females)	+ *				

* = 0.05; ** = 0.01; *** = 0.001; + *** positive; − ** negative.
PWS: Prader–Willi syndrome; LD: learning disabilities.

delay of the PWS group compared with the LD group, and the correlations with IQ were expected.

Factor analysis was carried out for the reported behaviours, separately for the PWS and LD groups. In the factor analysis for the PWS group, three factors emerged. These, together with factor loadings, are presented in Table 8.10. These factors

Table 8.8. Correlates of age, IQ, severity of eating disorder and current Body Mass Index (BMI) with behaviour checklists and adaptive behaviour domain standard scores

	Children	PWS	LD	Adults	PWS	LD
Age	DBC full scale score	+ *	− *	ABC full scale score	+ ***	− **
	Anxiety scale		− *	Irritability scale	+ **	
	Autistic traits scale	+ **		Lethargy scale	+ ***	− *
IQ	Antisocial scale		+ **	ABC full scale score	− **	
				Irritability scale	− ***	
				Lethargy scale	− *	
				Stereotypy scale	− *	− *
				Inappropriate speech	− **	
Eating	DBC full scale score	+ **	+ **	Hyperactivity scale	+ *	
	Disruptive scale	+ **	+ **			
	Self absorbed scale		+ *			
	Communication scale	+ *				
	Anxiety scale		+ **			
	Antisocial scale	+ ***	+ **			

Adaptive Behaviour Domain Standard Scores	Children		Adults		All	
	PWS	LD	PWS	LD	PWS	LD
Age						
Communication	− ***				− ***	− *
Daily living skills	− ***		− **		− ***	
Socialisation	− ***		− **		− ***	− *
Maladaptive behaviour			+ ***		− ***	− **
IQ						
Communication	+ ***	+ *	+ ***	+ ***	+ ***	+ ***
Daily living skills	+ **		+ ***	+ ***	+ ***	+ ***
Socialisation	+ *		+ ***	+ ***	+ **	+ ***
Maladaptive behaviour			− *		− *	
Eating						
Communication					− **	
Socialisation	− *				− ***	
Maladaptive behaviour	+ ***	+ ***		+ **		+ ***
BMI						
Communication	− *		+ *		− ***	
Daily living skills				+ **		
Socialisation	− *				− **	
Maladaptive behaviour					+ *	+ *

DBC: Development Behaviour Checklist; ABC: Aberrant Behaviour Checklist; PWS: Prader–Willi syndrome; LD: learning disabilities.

Table 8.9. Correlates of age, IQ, severity of eating disorder and current Body Mass Index (BMI) with adaptive behaviour sub-domain age equivalents

Sub-domain age scores		Children		Adults		All	
		PWS	LD	PWS	LD	PWS	LD
Age	Receptive	+ ***	+ ***			+ ***	
	Expressive	+ ***	+ ***	− *		+ **	
	Written	+ ***	+ ***			+ ***	
	Personal	+ ***	+ ***	− **		+ ***	+ *
	Domestic	+ ***	+ ***			+ ***	+ ***
	Community	+ ***	+ ***	− *		+ ***	+ **
	Interpersonal	+ ***	+ ***	− *		+ ***	
	Play & leisure	+ ***	+ ***	− ***		+ **	+ *
	Coping		+ ***	− *		+ ***	+ ***
IQ	Receptive			+ ***	+ ***	+ ***	+ **
	Expressive	+ **	+ ***	+ ***	+ ***	+ ***	+ ***
	Written	+ ***	+ **	+ ***	+ ***	+ ***	+ ***
	Personal			+ ***	+ ***	+ ***	+ **
	Domestic	+ *		+ **	+ ***	+ ***	+ **
	Community	+ *	+ ***	+ ***	+ ***	+ ***	
	Interpersonal			+ ***	+ **	+ ***	+ **
	Play & leisure	+ *	+ *	+ ***	+ ***	+ ***	+ ***
	Coping			+ ***	+ ***	+ *	
Eating	Domestic	− *					+ *
	Community					+ *	
	Interpersonal					+ *	
	Coping	− **					− **
BMI	Receptive	+ *					+ **
	Expressive	+ *	+ *		+ **		+ **
	Written	+ *	+ *				+ *
	Personal	+ ***	+ *			+ *	+ **
	Domestic	+ **		+ **		+ *	+ ***
	Community	+ ***	+ *		+ *	+ **	+ ***
	Interpersonal	+ ***			+ *	+ **	+ *
	Play & leisure	+ ***				+ **	
	Coping	+ *					

PWS: Prader–Willi syndrome; LD: learning disabilities.

Table 8.10. Factor analyses of behaviours in Prader–Willi syndrome (PWS) and learning disabilities (LD) groups

PWS factor analysis					
FACTOR 1: eating		FACTOR 2: personality		FACTOR 3: emotions	
Eating behaviour	0.82	Obsessive	0.58	Mood swings	0.50
Lying	0.88	Temper tantrums	0.73	Skin picking	0.68
Stealing	0.75	Possessive	0.69	Stubborn	0.75
		Violent/aggressive	0.68	Argumentative	0.64
		Repetitive questions	0.49		
LD factor analysis					
FACTOR 1: eating		FACTOR 2: aggression		FACTOR 3:	
Eating behaviour	0.78	Skin picking	0.81	Repetitive questions	0.94
Lying	0.90	Temper tantrums	0.71	Possessive	0.79
Stealing	0.67	Argumentative	0.73		
Mood swings	0.79	Violent/aggressive	0.68		
		Stubborn	0.64		
FACTOR 4:					
Obsessive	0.90				

roughly correspond to eating, personality and emotions, as discussed below. For the comparison LD group, four factors emerged in the factor analysis. These, together with factor loadings, are also presented in Table 8.10. In PWS, *eating behaviour* is a separate factor from *temper tantrums, obsessiveness, mood swings* and other maladaptive behaviours, indicating that its genetic and neurobiological basis may be different from these other behaviours. The independence of eating behaviour from other characteristic PWS behaviours may be indicative of a specific pathophysiological mechanism and might account for the failure of satiation, which has been proposed to be the basis for the over-eating behaviour in PWS.[17]

The strength of the Cambridge study is the fact that it is population-based, and therefore relatively free from referral bias. However, few details were available for those who did not volunteer for the full phenotype study (see Chapter 3), and those that volunteered for the population-based study may be different in important respects. Thus, this study went as far as possible to eliminate potential biases of this kind, but cannot rule them out completely. The study included a matched comparison group. There has been much debate in the behavioural phenotype literature as to the best comparison group.[15, 19] We amalgamated two groups: (1) those who volunteered and were thought to have PWS, but were found not to have the full clinical features or the PWS genotype; and (2) children and adults identified through a local special school and social services provision, respectively. The advantage of such a group was that it was not made up of people with one single syndrome who, because of the characteristics of that syndrome, may have distorted any comparison. In addition, a proportion were also obese, and there was a sufficient range of *BMI* in the comparison group to enable us to examine a relationship between behaviour and *BMI* in that group, as well as in those with PWS.

In this first population-based study there is further evidence for a distinctive behavioural phenotype in PWS. The range and nature of behaviours that occur in excess are consistent with findings from other studies.[14, 15, 18, 27, 28] The key diagnostic characteristics and all the 'behavioural' characteristics assessed, except possessiveness, lying and argumentativeness, were found to be significantly more prevalent among those with PWS. In addition to the eating disorder, which was almost universal, temper tantrums, skin picking, mood fluctuations, repetitive questioning and obsessional traits were among the most prevalent of behavioural characteristics. We concluded that the comparative low prevalence rates in the comparison group indicated that these behaviours were not associated with an 'obesity syndrome', or with the presence of a learning disability. Thus, one effect of the PWS genotype is an increased propensity to these specific behaviours.

The findings on the informant child and adult questionnaires were more equivocal. The Development Behaviour Checklist scores in the children did not significantly differ between the groups, although average scores exceeded 1 in the PWS group on items relating to obsessiveness, peer relationships and skin picking. In adults, the full scale scores and scores on the Irritability Sub-scale of the Aberrant Behaviour Checklist were higher in the PWS group, and in the maladaptive behaviour scale of the Vineland Adaptive Behaviour Scales, scores were also higher (both children and adults).

An examination of the relationship between these behavioural variables and age, IQ, severity of eating disorder and current *BMI* revealed that in both groups increasing age was associated with a high *BMI* and, in the PWS group, also with severity of the eating disorder. These findings are likely to be explained by increasing independence from parental control and, in the PWS group, possibly by the later diagnosis of the older group. Aberrant behaviour increased with age in the PWS group, but decreased in the LD group. It decreased with increased IQ in PWS adults. In both groups, over-eating was associated with more aberrant behaviour. Adaptive behaviours showed that the PWS group was stronger on Daily Living Skills and weaker on Socialisation, compared with the LD group. There were relative strengths in the Community sub-domain, and a relative weakness in the Coping Skills sub-domain, although these were not statistically significant.

We looked at clustering of behavioural variables in PWS and the LD group to investigate possible common mechanisms in their occurrence. When the behavioural data was analysed using factor analysis, the three factors made intuitive sense in the context of PWS, and agreed with evidence given to us by parents and other carers, and with observations in the literature. The first factor extracted consisted of the severity of the eating behaviour, lying and stealing. The lying and stealing by many people with PWS is solely, or mainly, associated with food (or money to buy food), and in many cases confined to home. We found that many people with the syndrome do not lie about issues less salient to their own priorities. Like hypotonia and hypogonadism, the eating disorder is almost universal, and is not invariably associated with other PWS behaviours.

The second factor extracted consisted of obsessive behaviour, temper tantrums, violent/aggressive behaviour and possessiveness. Our hypothesis was that such behaviours have a common aetiology in developmental delay, which provides the biological basis for such behaviour, with environmental influences modifying its precise form and content. For example, many parents saw temper tantrums as being provoked more by the thwarting of obsessive behaviour than by pure food issues.[28] Frequently the two are confounded – a meal is late or a promised food treat has to be cancelled or postponed – but many parents believed that it was the not keeping to schedule or apparent breaking of a promise that is the real issue, and that similar outbursts arose when transport was late or an outing had to be cancelled. Aggressive or violent behaviour was almost always reported as 'only in tantrums', so the finding that these load on the same factor was expected.

The third factor extracted links together mood swings, skin picking and argumentativeness. This, too, makes sense in the context of PWS, and in our interviews with parents and carers they have remarked on deteriorating behaviour associated with low mood. At a UK PWSA meeting some young people with PWS spoke about what the syndrome meant to them. One described the bullying and ridicule endured at school, and the resulting decision to stop trying to curb eating and 'eat myself to death'. Although a single, anecdotal and extreme instance, this does illustrate how low mood and self-injurious behaviour might be linked, especially when access to food is limited by vigilant carers.

The LD group may or may not have been typical of people with LD, in that a good proportion were overweight and very interested in food (average *BMIs* in the two groups were 31.0 PWS and 28.7 LD and maximum mean *BMIs* in those over 16 years were 43.8 and 39.4 respectively). Again, lying and stealing were associated with food, but so also was mood. It seems, in this group, that eating behaviour and mood share a common basis. This relationship has also been shown in studies of the effect of dieting on 5-HT receptor function and mood.[29] In this group there also seemed to be a factor of pure aggression, including both aggression to the self and to others, and unlike PWS, this appeared to have nothing to do with obsessive behaviour. Indeed, the latter was a separate factor in this LD group. The differences would suggest that there are likely to be differences between the two groups in terms of the neurobiological basis for, and aetiology of, these behaviours.

Explanatory models

Earlier in this Chapter, we proposed three putative explanatory models that could explain the relationship between a particular genetic syndrome and cognitive function and behaviour. How might they account for what is observed in PWS? Given the universality of the eating disorder in PWS, we propose that for this behaviour the 'all or nothing' model applies. We predict that there is a direct relationship between the abnormal expression of a specific gene in the PWS critical region and eating behaviour. A useful model for such a relationship is the ob/ob mice,[30] and the reports of leptin, and leptin receptor abnormalities, and the beneficial effects of leptin replacement in the former group, associated with single gene mutations in families.[31,32,33] In these families it is presumed that it is the failure of feedback mechanisms that leads to excessive eating and to extreme obesity. Whilst there is no evidence of a leptin, or leptin receptor abnormalities in PWS, we think it is likely that an analogous mechanism, probably involving a central neurotransmitter/receptor system, will eventually be found to be present. Given the characteristic presence of short stature and delayed sexual development in PWS, we propose that the site of action is likely to be in the hypothalamus. Swaab et al.,[34] in a study of hypothalamic tissue from five brains from people with PWS, have reported a reduction in oxytocin levels in the paraventricular hypothalamic nucleus, and they have proposed that this might account for the abnormal satiety response to food intake. More recently Goldstone et al. have reported low, rather than the predicted high, levels of neuropeptide Y.[35]

We have argued elsewhere (see Chapter 11) that the obsessive–compulsive behaviours observed in PWS are best conceptualised as a consequence of arrested brain development, rather than a true obsessive–compulsive disorder.[16] As was proposed there, we believe that our data support this view. The rates of such behaviour do not change significantly with age, they are present from early childhood, and have similar characteristics to the normal obsessive behaviours found in children.[36,37] The factor analysis gives indirect support to this view as obsessive–compulsive behaviour was separate from skin picking and moodiness, and therefore we propose they do not share a similar neurobiological basis. Similarly we hypothesise that the propensity to temper tantrums is best conceptualised in a similar manner. Arrested development results in a continuing propensity to such behaviours throughout life, with disruption of routine being the trigger for such behaviour. Support for this comes from the fact that temper tantrums are negatively correlated with ability, suggesting that some people with PWS do develop sufficiently to move beyond that developmental stage, and to acquire better coping skills. The fact that obsessional behaviours and temper tantrums are not universal could be explained by differential influences on development and the stage of developmental arrest.

Dimitropoulos *et al.*[22] investigated this developmental perspective by examining the age of onset of such behaviours in children with Down syndrome (DS), PWS, and a 'typically developing' comparison group. They observed that the number of compulsive behaviours were not significantly different between a typically developing group and those with PWS at ages 2–3 years, but were different at ages 4–6 years. This gives some support to the view that normal obsessive–compulsive behaviours appear in young children with PWS, but the abnormality is that such behaviours persist. Their study also illustrates the problem of a DS control group, as the young DS group were less compulsive than the typically developing children, and therefore atypical in the opposite direction to PWS. We therefore propose that one action of the PWS genotype is to lead to a specific pattern of atypical and arrested brain development such that the characteristic rituals and compulsions of early childhood continue, and only resolve if development goes beyond that particular developmental phase.

The cognitive findings, discussed in Chapter 7, showed that in the population-based sample there is a normal distribution of scores with a mean of about 60. We do not have data on parental ability, but have put forward the hypothesis that this is an example of a shift in threshold, resulting in a greater proportion of the group falling into the learning disabled range. We would predict that the shift in IQ for the group as a whole is due to a major effect of a single gene, with polygenic and environmental factors accounting for the distribution of scores within the group.

One very striking finding,[20] discussed in Chapter 10, is that those with chromosome 15 disomies all developed a severe affective psychotic illness by the time they had reached early adult life. This was not true for those with chromosome 15 deletions. This finding would suggest that it is not PWS per se that carries an increased risk of psychotic illness, but rather the maternal disomy 15. We have proposed that the effect on the expression of maternally and paternally imprinted genes of having a maternal chromosome 15 disomy is a likely explanation of this finding. As is the case with the eating disorder, the fact that it is universal in those with disomy would suggest that there is a direct relationship between gene expression and the development of psychotic illness. Interestingly, mood swings were reported among those with disomy and deletions, and clustered with skin picking and stubbornness. These behaviours were independent of the risk of psychotic illness and, we speculate, may represent a threshold change. If this is the case, it might correlate with parental personality traits. Investigation of correlations with a family history of these would clarify whether this is the correct conceptual model. A recent paper, looking at gene expression in deletion and disomy subtypes of PWS, may be relevant to our findings regarding (short-term) mood swings and psychotic illness. Expression at GABRA3 and GABRA5 in disomy PWS was intermediate in strength between those of deletions and normals, while expression of the maternally expressed UBE3A and ATP10C in disomies was double those of both deletions and normals.[38]

We speculate that the three factors extracted in the factor analysis have a different neurobiological basis, and might correspond to the failure of expression of different imprinted genes in the PWS critical region. This can only be tested as the genotype of PWS becomes clearer but, if these proposed models are correct, the genotype of PWS must be able to account for the varying manifestations of the behaviours described. In rare genetic syndromes involving a single gene, such as Lesch–Nyhan and Rett syndromes, the behavioural phenotype can be characterised in terms of one major disturbance (self-injurious behaviour and regression in development from early childhood, respectively). The 'all or none' model is most appropriate in these cases: the behaviour is always observed. In contrast, PWS and Williams syndrome (deletion of about 1.5 Megabases on chromosome 7) are thought to involve multiple genes, and have complex behavioural phenotypes, with at least some characteristics that are not universal. In these cases, more than one of our models may be appropriate. The complexity of the PWS phenotype may therefore result from the action of different genes that have direct or indirect effects on manifest behaviours, early development and cognitive function.

REFERENCES

1. Nyhan, W. L. Forward. In O'Brien, G. & Yule, W. (Eds). *Behavioral Phenotypes*. London: MacKeith Press, 1995.
2. Flint, J. & Yule, W. Behavioural phenotypes. In Rutter, M., Taylor, E. & Hersov, L. (Eds). *Child and Adolescent Psychiatry: Modern Approaches*. London: Blackwell Scientific, 1994.
3. Turk, J. & Hill, P. Behavioural phenotypes in dysmorphic syndromes. *Clinical Dysmorphology* **4** (1995), 105–115.
4. O'Brien, G. & Yule, W. Why behavioral phenotypes. In O'Brien, G. & Yule, W. (Eds). *Behavioral Phenotypes*. London: MacKeith Press, 1995.
5. Flint, J. Annotation: behavioural phenotypes: a window onto the biology of behaviour. *Journal of Child Psychology and Psychiatry* **37** (1996), 355–367.
6. Verkerk, A. J., Pieretti, M., Sutcliffe, J. S. *et al.* Identification of a gene (FMR-1) containing a CGG repeat coincident with a breakpoint cluster region exhibiting length variation in fragile X syndrome. *Cell* **65** (1991), 905–914.
7. Hodapp, R. M. Direct and indirect behavioural effects of different genetic disorders of mental retardation. *American Journal on Mental Retardation* **102** (1997), 67–79.
8. Plomin, R. & Rutter, M. Child development, molecular genetics, and what to do with genes once they are found. *Child Development* **69** (1998), 1223–1242.

9. Hodapp, R. M. & Dykens, E. M. Strengthening behavioural phenotype research on genetic mental retardation syndromes. *American Journal on Mental Retardation* **106** (2001), 4–15.

10. Lefebvre, L., Viville, S., Barton, S. C., Ishino, F., Keverne, E. B. & Surani, M. A. Abnormal maternal behaviour and growth retardation associated with loss of the imprinted gene MEST. *Nature Genetics* **20** (1998), 163–169.

11. Udwin, O. & Yule, W. A cognitive and behavioural phenotype in Williams syndrome. *Journal of Clinical and Experimental Neuropsychology* **13** (1991), 232–244.

12. Karmiloff-Smith, A., Grant, J., Berthoud, I., Davies, M., Howlin, P. & Udwin, O. Language and Williams syndrome: how intact is 'intact'? *Child Development* **68** (1997), 246–262.

13. Rubinsztein, J. S., Rubinsztein, D. C., Goodburn, S. & Holland, A. J. Apathy and hypersomnia are common features of myotonic dystrophy. *Journal of Neurology, Neurosurgery and Psychiatry* **64** (1998), 510–515.

14. Clarke, D. J., Boer, H., Chung, M. C., Sturmey, P. & Webb, T. Maladaptive behaviour in Prader–Willi syndrome in adult life. *Journal of Intellectual Disability Research* **40** (1996), 159–165.

15. Dykens, E. M. & Kasari, C. Maladaptive behavior in children with Prader–Willi syndrome, Down syndrome, and nonspecific Mental Retardation. *American Journal on Mental Retardation* **102** (1997), 228–237.

16. Clarke, D. J., Boer, H., Whittington, J. E., Holland, A. J., Butler, J. V. & Webb, T. Prader–Willi syndrome, compulsive and ritualistic behaviours: the first population-based survey. *British Journal of Psychiatry* **180** (2002), 358–362.

17. Holland, A. J., Treasure, J., Coskeran, P., Dallow, J., Milton, N. & Hillhouse, E. Measurement of excessive appetite and metabolic changes in Prader–Willi syndrome. *International Journal of Obesity* **17** (1993), 526–532.

18. Dykens, E. M., Hodapp, R. M., Walsh, K. & Nash, L. J. Adaptive and maladaptive behavior in Prader–Willi syndrome. *Journal of the American Academy of Child and Adolescent Psychiatry* **31** (1992), 1131–1135.

19. Dykens, E. M., Cassidy, S. B. & King, B. H. Maladaptive behavior differences in Prader–Willi syndrome due to paternal deletion versus maternal uniparental disomy. *American Journal on Mental Retardation* **104** (1999), 67–77.

20. Boer, H., Holland, A. J., Whittington, J. E., Butler, J. V., Webb, T. & Clarke, D. J. Psychotic illness in people with Prader–Willi syndrome due to chromosome 15 maternal uniparental disomy. *Lancet* **359** (2002), 135–136.

21. Holland, A. J., Whittington, J. E., Webb, T., Butler, J. V., Clarke, D. J. & Boer, H. Investigating brain function and behaviour in Prader–Willi syndrome. Paper presented at the *4th Triennial IPWSO Scientific Conference 2001, Saint Paul, Minnesota, USA*.

22. Dimitropoulos, A., Feurer, I. D., Butler, M. G. & Thompson, T. Emergence of compulsive behavior and tantrums in children with Prader–Willi syndrome. *American Journal of Mental Retardation* **106** (2001), 39–51.

23. Einfeld, S. & Tonge, B. J. *Developmental Behaviour Checklist – Parental version*. Clayton Australia: Centre for Developmental Psychiatry, 1989.

24. Aman, M. G., Singh, N. N., Stewart, A. W. *et al. Aberrant Behavior Checklist*. New York: Slosson, 1986.

25. Wechsler, D. *Intelligence and Attainment Scales – WAIS, WISC, WPPSI, WORD, WOND, WOLD.* Psychological Corporation. London: Harcourt Brace & Co. 1993.

26. Sparrow, S. S., Balla, D. A. & Cicchetti, D. V. *Vineland Adaptive Behavior Scales.* Windsor: NFER-Nelson, 1984.

27. Dykens, E. M. & Cassidy, S. B. Correlates of maladaptive behavior in children and adults with Prader–Willi syndrome. *American Journal of Medical Genetics (Neuropsychiatric Genetics)* **60** (1995), 546–549.

28. Dykens, E. M., Leckman, J. F. & Cassidy, S. B. Obsessions and compulsions in Prader–Willi syndrome. *Journal of Child Psychology and Psychiatry* **37** (1996), 995–1002.

29. Cowen, P. J., Clifford, E. M., Walsh, A. E. S., Williams, C. & Fairburn, C. G. Moderate dieting causes 5-HT$_{2c}$ receptor supersensitivity. *Psychological Medicine* **26** (1996), 1155–1159.

30. Samad, F. & Loskutoff, D. J. The fat mouse: a powerful genetic model to study elevated plasminogen activator inhibitor 1 in obesity/NIDDM. *Thrombosis and Haemostasis* **78** (1997), 652–655.

31. Montague, C. T., Farooqi, I. S., Whitehead, J. P. *et al.* Congenital leptin deficiency is associated with severe early-onset obesity in humans. *Nature* **387** (1997), 903–908.

32. Farooqi, I. S., Jebb, S. A., Langmack, G. *et al.* Effects of recombinant leptin therapy in a child with congenital leptin deficiency. *New England Journal of Medicine* **341** (1999), 879–884.

33. O'Rahilly, S. Life without leptin. *Nature* **392** (1998), 330–331.

34. Swaab, D. F., Purba, J. S. & Hofman, M. A. Alterations in the hypothalamic paraventricular nucleus and its oxytocin neurons (putative satiety cells) in Prader–Willi syndrome: a study of five cases. *Journal of Clinical Endocrinology and Metabolism* **80** (1995), 573–579.

35. Goldstone, A. P., Thomas, E. L., Brynes, A. E. *et al.* Visceral adipose tissue and metabolic complications of obesity are reduced in Prader–Willi syndrome female adults: evidence for novel influences on body fat distribution. *Journal of Clinical Endocrinology and Metabolism* **86** (2001), 4330–4338.

36. Evans, D. W., Leckman, J. F., Carter, A. *et al.* Ritual, habit and perfectionism: the prevalence and development of compulsive-like behavior in normal young children. *Child Development* **68** (1997), 56–68.

37. Zohar, A. H. & Bruno, R. Normative and pathological obsessive–compulsive behavior and ideation in childhood: a question of timing. *Journal of Child Psychology and Psychiatry* **38** (1997), 993–999.

38. Bittel, D. C., Kibiryeva, N., Talebizadeh, Z. & Butler, M. G. Microarray analysis of gene/transcript expression in Prader–Willi syndrome: deletion versus UPD. *Journal of Medical Genetics* **40** (2003), 568–574.

9

Medical conditions affecting people with PWS

As we noted in Chapters 1 and 3, few older people with PWS have been reported in the literature and in our population-based cohort no one was identified older than 46 years of age at the standardisation date, the turn of the twenty-first century. We estimated a birth incidence for PWS of 1:22 000 and a population prevalence of no less than 1:52 000, with a mortality rate of about three per cent per year. Some support for the interpretation of our findings, of a more or less constant mortality rate across ages, has come from a report on sudden death of people with PWS in Australia, which found mortality among all age groups (see Chapter 4). Previous reports indicated that the most common cause of death was cor pulmonale possibly attributable to severe obesity.[1] Also the neonatal hypotonia is thought to contribute to the presence of strabismus, scoliosis and respiratory problems in children, and the obesity to non-insulin dependent diabetes mellitus (NIDDM) and heart conditions in older people.[2]

This chapter describes the prevalence rates of physical morbidity in the population-based cohort of children and adults with the syndrome, and we argue that some are a direct and others a secondary consequence of the syndrome. The aim is to determine what might account for the high mortality rate, and thereby aid the development of preventative treatment strategies.

The semi-structured interview with families or carers of people with PWS (Chapter 3, Appendix 3.1) included questions about physical health problems experienced over the participant's lifetime, with specific reference to those conditions considered to be associated with PWS: diabetes; heart problems; scoliosis; strabismus; recurrent respiratory problems; hypogonadism; and sleep disorders.[3,4,5,6] Report of a health problem led to further inquiry as to age of onset and treatment. No physical examinations were carried out, apart from recordings of current height and weight. Maximum lifetime weight was documented, when known.

To facilitate further study of the causation of health problems, the population cohort was expanded by inclusion of volunteers diagnosed with PWS, but who were residing or originating from outside the health region. The findings are based on a

Table 9.1. Details of Prader–Willi syndrome cohort studied

	Population sample	Volunteers from outside region	Total cohort
No. in study (m:f)	66 (40:26)	42 (20:22)	108 (60:48)
No. >17yr (m:f)	32 (20:12)	26 (12:14)	58 (32:26)
No. <18yr (m:f)	34 (20:14)	16 (8:8)	50 (28: 22)
Mean Age	19.0 yr (SD 12.9)	18.3 (SD 9.6)	18.7 yr (SD 11.7)
Mean BMI(>17 yr)	37.4 (SD 12.4, $n = 30$)	31.7 (SD 10.3, $n = 25$)	34.8 (SD 11.8, $n = 55$)
Mean BMI (<18 yr)	26.6 (SD 9.885, $n = 28$)	23.5 (SD 6.5, $n = 15$)	25.5 (SD 8.9, $n = 43$)
Mean IQ	61.0 (SD 13.2, $n = 56$)	66.8 (SD 8.4, $n = 38$)	63.4 (SD 11.8, $n = 94$)

m: male; f: female; BMI: Body Mass Index.

group of 108 (66 in the population-based sample, and 42 from outside) individuals, age range 0–46 years, who either had a genetic diagnosis of PWS or who did not give a blood sample but met clinical diagnostic criteria. Details of these participants are given in Table 9.1. Prevalence rates in the text refer to the population sample but, as rates were similar in the expanded cohort, the latter were used to investigate possible aetiological factors for each disorder. Because of the small numbers for each disorder and the large standard deviation found when calculating mean values, statistical evaluation was not always appropriate. A summary of the reports of medical conditions are shown in Table 9.2.

This study has identified a particular profile of physical morbidity that affects people with PWS. This includes NIDDM, recurrent respiratory infections, scoliosis and sleep disorders, and to a lesser extent, hypertension and leg ulceration. Osteo-porosis may also be common. The findings on the components of this profile of physical morbidity are presented and discussed below.

Non-insulin dependent diabetes mellitus (NIDDM)

Descriptive details from the diabetic and non-diabetic groups in the expanded cohort are shown in Table 9.3. At the time of interview, four of the 15 with diabetes required insulin. However, all had had their diabetes controlled by diet or oral agents alone for some periods of time, and six of the 15 linked diminishing medication requirements to weight loss.

NIDDM was once considered to be so frequent in PWS that early papers included it as one of the primary features.[7] Our findings (Table 9.2) showed that it still greatly exceeds the 1–5% quoted for the general population, or 6–20% in obese caucasian adults,[8,9,10,11,12] where the risk doubles with every 20% of excess weight.[13] The mean Body Mass Index (BMI) of participants was above the accepted normal value

Table 9.2. Prevalence of medical conditions in the Prader–Willi syndrome population sample and the expanded cohort

Condition (lifetime history)	Prevalence					
	Under 18 years		Over 17 years		All ages	
	population sample (%)	expanded cohort (%)	population sample (%)	expanded cohort (%)	population sample (%)	expanded cohort (%)
NIDDM (non-insulin dependent diabetes mellitus)	**0/34**	1/50 (2)	**8/32 (25)**	14/58 (24)	**8/66 (12)**	15/108 (14)
Hypertension	**0/34**	0/50	**2/31 (6)**	7/56 (13)	**2/65 (3)**	7/106 (7)
Other diagnosed cardiac illness	**0/34**	0/50	**2/32 (6)**	2/57 (3)	**2/66 (3)**	2/107 (2)
Reported serious leg oedema/ulceration	**0/34**	0/50	**7/32 (22)**	12/58 (21)	**7/66 (11)**	12/108 (11)
Recurrent respiratory problems	**18/34 (53)**	24/50 (48)	**12/32 (38)**	21/57 (37)	**30/66 (46)**	45/107 (42)
Respiratory illness requiring hospital treatment	–	–	–	–	**10/65 (15)**	16/106 (15)
Total suspected scoliosis/kyphosis	**10/34 (29)**	17/50 (34)	**12/31 (39)**	23/56 (41)	**22/65 (34)**	40/106 (38)
Numbers where scoliosis observed by a professional	**9/34 (26)**	14/50 (28)	**10/31 (32)**	19/56 (34)	**19/65 (29)**	33/106 (31)
Scoliosis-numbers where serious deformity/ intervention	**5/34 (15)**	7/50 (14)	**5/31 (16)**	7/56 (13)	**10/65 (15)**	14/106 (13)
Confirmed osteoporosis	–	–	–	1/58 (2)	–	1/108 (1)
History of any fracture	**7/34 (21)**	8/50 (16)	**12/32 (38)**	25/58 (43)	**19/66 (29)**	33/108 (31)
male	**5/20 (25)**	5/28 (18)	**8/20 (40)**	15/32 (47)	**13/40 (33)**	20/60 (33)
female	**2/14 (14)**	3/22 (14)	**4/12 (33)**	10/26 (38)	**6/26 (23)**	13/48 (27)
History of >1 fracture	**1/34 (3)**	2/50 (4)	**7/32 (22)**	13/58 (22)	**8/66 (12)**	15/108 (14)
male	–	–	**5/20 (25)**	8/32 (25)	**5/40 (13)**	8/60 (13)
female	**1/14 (7)**	2/22 (9)	**2/12 (17)**	5/26 (19)	**3/26 (12)**	7/48 (15)
Strabismus	**20/34 (59)**	27/50 (54)	**18/30 (60)**	32/54 (59)	**38/64 (59)**	59/104 (57)
(undergone surgery)	**5/20 (25)**	7/27 (26)	**5/18 (28)**	12/32 (37)	**10/38 (26)**	19/59 (32)

Table 9.3. Diabetes mellitus: descriptive details from the expanded Prader–Willi syndrome (PWS) cohort

	Non-diabetic PWS over 13 years[a] (*n*)	PWS with diabetes (*n*)
Mean age of cohort	25.3 yr SD 8.3 (53)	28.5 yr SD 7.6 (15)
Mean age at onset of diabetes	–	20.5 yr SD 8.2 (14)
Mean age at start of obesity problems	4.0 yr SD 3.5 (49)	4.4 yr SD 5.0 (14)
Mean age at heaviest	20.9 yr SD 5.9 (51)	24.7 yr SD 8.1 (15)
Mean BMI in kg/m^2	34.1 SD 12.2 (49)	37.0 SD 10.0 (15)
Mean max BMI in kg/m^{2b}	42.1 SD 13.4 (42)	48.0 SD 19.6 (14)
Number experiencing serious leg oedema ± ulcers	8/53 (15%)	4/15 (27%) (2 MRSA carriers)
Number with history of hypertension	2/53 (4%)	5/15 (30%)[c]
Gender ratio, m:f	31:22	7:8
Positive family history (In first or second degree relatives).	7/53 (13%)	4/13 (31%)

[a] age of youngest person with non-insulin dependent diabetes mellitus in expanded cohort was 14 years.

[b] Calculated only for adults over 17 years where height known.

[c] ($P < 0.01$).

MRSA: methicillin-resistant *Staphylococcus aureus*.

of 20–25 kg/m^2 (see Tables 9.1 and 9.3) and, while BMI at the onset of NIDDM was unknown, the mean *maximum adult lifetime BMI* in the diabetic group was slightly, though not significantly, higher than in the non-diabetic group. In the general population, NIDDM is uncommon under 30 years although this is changing as rates of obesity increase.[11, 13] The early onset in PWS may, as has been suggested in non-PWS populations,[10, 13, 14] be related to the duration of the weight problems that begin in childhood (Table 9.3). Increased occurrence of adolescent NIDDM in the general population has been reported in association with rising levels of obesity.[15] There may be other risk factors typical of PWS, such as the truncal distribution of fat or low activity levels,[13, 16, 17] that combine to give rise to early onset of NIDDM. Literature reports on differences in glucose and insulin metabolism in PWS are conflicting.[2, 9] As in the general population, a *positive family history* was more frequent in those with NIDDM (Table 9.3), but this was not statistically significant.

The reported relationship between weight and medication reinforces, as in the non-PWS population,[13, 14] the importance of weight control in the management and possible prevention of NIDDM and subsequent related morbidity. Truncal obesity correlates with diabetes and hypertension in the general population.[13, 18] Morbidity with respect to hypertension was noted to be significantly increased in the diabetic group and problems with leg ulceration were also more common.

We concluded that there are likely to be several risk factors for the development of NIDDM in people with PWS, including early onset and prolonged obesity, low levels of activity, the distribution of weight and a positive family history of NIDDM, some of which are preventable.

Cardiovascular disorders

Few clearly diagnosed cardiovascular problems were reported (see Table 9.2). This concurs with the literature on PWS that has few examples of reported pre-mortem coronary artery disease, Lamb & Johnson[4] citing one of the few cases. The reported prevalence of hypertension in our population-based cohort appeared low compared with previous studies.[19] Only four people with PWS were currently being treated with medication; the others had responded to weight reduction. The prevalence was only very slightly raised compared to that found in the general population, where approximately 1.4% of the 18- to 49-year-old age group receive medication for hypertension, while a further 2.5% have untreated hypertension greater than 160/90 mmHg.[8] Rabkin et al.[11] reported a trebling in rates of hypertension among adults in the general population with a BMI of greater than 30 kg/m^2, compared with those of normal weight. The influence of weight was most marked in younger age groups, where 18% of such obese adults aged under 35 years had blood pressure greater than 140/90 mmHg, compared with 3% of their normal weight peers. These figures would appear to indicate that, in the PWS population, possibly excluding those with NIDDM, individuals are less susceptible to hypertension than one might expect from their weight. As we relied on self-report data, it is possible that our findings were an under-representation, as blood pressure may not have been being fully monitored.

Respiratory disorders

Respiratory histories did not always distinguish between asthma and bronchitis. In our study, all instances where carers recollected periods when recurrent respiratory illness had been a 'notable problem' were included (see Table 9.2). The mean *age of onset* of problems in the expanded cohort was 1.7 years (sd 4.2, $n = 39$), with a smaller proportion, (9/58,15%), continuing with recurrent problems in adulthood. Five adults (9%) and 10 under-18-year-olds (20%) had a *current prescription* for bronchodilators or steroids.

The inclusion of all respiratory illness together, because of problems obtaining detailed histories, made it difficult to compare directly with the general population. The apparent decline in lifetime prevalence in adults may be a result of sample error. Well-informed parents, sensitive to the risk of respiratory problems in their offspring, may over-report, whereas, in older people with PWS, such illnesses would be less likely to be remembered retrospectively unless severe. However, rates do appear high. Childhood respiratory illness in the general population is thought to be associated with adult respiratory morbidity, possibly due to an underlying predisposition or the resultant lung damage.[20] This, in itself, could explain the adult rates of illness found, although one might have expected increasing weight and low activity to have further compromised pulmonary function. The predominance of symptoms in early childhood supports previous findings that hypotonia, persisting into and often beyond, infancy is implicated in the reduction of pulmonary function and increased susceptibility to infection.[6] In addition, most babies with PWS are unable to breast feed and miss the initial protective immunological benefit of breast milk in very early life.

Scoliosis

Figures for scoliosis are shown in Table 9.2. Females with PWS were at greater risk of scoliosis than males, the ratio being 1.23:1, increasing to 2.3:1 for those with severe deformity. From the expanded cohort, it was noted that the initial diagnosis was made in childhood (mean age 7.7 years, SD 6.8, $n = 34$), with varying degrees of progression in later life. In eight female participants, problems were not noted until the early teens and, of these, four progressed rapidly. The *mean* BMI of those with reported scoliosis (29.9 kg/m^2, SD 11.8, $n = 34$) and those without (31.2 kg/m^2, SD 11.5, $n = 61$), were not significantly different. In at least 22/40 (55%), and in 11/15 (79%) of those classed as severe, scoliosis was first noted prior to any excessive weight gain. No significant difference in respiratory problems was detected between those with and those without a history of scoliosis.

The overall prevalence rate for reported scoliosis (see Table 9.2) was much higher than the 2–14% quoted for the general adolescent population,[21] but lower than in previous reports relating to PWS.[1,22] The male/female ratio concurs with findings in the general population, where females with idiopathic scoliosis outnumber males.[21] It has been suggested that scoliosis in PWS relates to hypotonia and obesity.[23] Hypotonia is probably a factor but is difficult to quantify retrospectively. The presence of obesity would seem less significant although it may play a part in the progression of the deformity. One participant reported that severe osteoporosis was discovered as an incidental finding during spinal surgery at 15 years. Other authors have also noted osteoporosis during surgery for scoliosis,[24] and questions have been raised about its role in the pathogenesis of the deformity.[25] In fact, the origins of idiopathic scoliosis are unclear. Disturbed feedback between proprioceptors in body and brain stem centres, visual/vestibular dysfunction and higher level CNS processing of vestibular information have all been implicated.[26] Poor balance and co-ordination was frequently mentioned as a feature of PWS by informants. This was not evaluated in this study. Intrinsic asymmetry, said to be common in PWS, in conjunction with low activity and poor tone, may also be a factor.[22] Scoliosis can be difficult to diagnose without X-ray examination, especially in overweight subjects,[22] and lesser deformities may have been under-reported. There seems to be no satisfactory way to predict in whom progression will occur, but it is thought most likely to occur during adolescence.[22,27] In this study, however, seven of the 14 participants with severe scoliosis had their first active intervention, including surgery, before the age of 10 years. Further progression frequently occurred during adolescence and six required operative treatment at that time. Although the chest deformity associated with scoliosis appears not to increase respiratory problems, prevention of deformity in PWS is important to avoid further jeopardizing mobility. With approximately 15% of the PWS population likely to develop severe problems, frequent monitoring is vital, particularly during early teenage years.

Osteoporosis

The only definitive diagnosis of osteoporosis reported in this study was outside the population sample. In the absence of bone density investigation, rates of bone fractures were explored and are reported in Table 9.2. However, osteoporosis is clearly associated with PWS.[25,28] Bone mineral content has been shown to be reduced in people with PWS and bone mineral density is reduced post-pubertally.[28] Our findings seem to indicate that, if problems exist, they are not being detected. This study did not examine bone density, but rates of reported fractures seemed high, although no comparative figures were available. From data in Table 9.2, it does appear that people with PWS continue to suffer fractures beyond the age of childhood accidents. There was no clear evidence that females were more predisposed to fracture than males; if anything the trend was the opposite. This is supported by reports from the recent International PWS conference of higher rates of osteoporosis in males.[29] In this study,[29] bone density determinations at the spine and at the femur showed that 39% and 53% of males and 14% and 16% of females had osteoporosis at these respective locations. Given the impairment of sex hormone release,[30] osteoporosis is likely and hormone replacement therapy is a reasonable preventative measure,[31] also inducing development of some secondary sex characteristics. However, the practice was not widespread in this population in either males or females. There are conflicting reports as to whether growth hormone significantly alters bone density, but it is reported to have other beneficial effects on body composition.[32,33,34,35] Relatively few individuals had been offered growth hormone and only two individuals had a current prescription for growth hormone.

Table 9.4. Prescription of hormones in the Prader–Willi syndrome population sample and the expanded cohort

	Prevalence					
	Under 18 years		Over 17 years		All ages	
Condition (lifetime history)	population sample (%)	expanded cohort (%)	population sample (%)	expanded cohort (%)	population sample (%)	expanded cohort (%)
Prescribed growth hormone	**4/34 (12)**	8/50 (16)	**3/31 (10)**	7/56 (13)	**7/65 (11)**	15/106 (14)
Prescribed sex hormone[a]	–	–	**11/41 (27)**	23/69 (33)	–	–
male[a]	–	–	**6/25 (24)**	11/37 (30)	–	–
female[a]	–	–	**5/16 (31)**	12/32 (38)	–	–

[a] Individuals aged 12 years and over.

Sexual development

Cryptorchidism (undescended or absent testes) was almost universal, occurring in 36/37 (97%) of males in the population sample, of whom 20 had undergone surgery. The other male in this sample also had abnormal sexual development, having such a small penis that normal male toilet use was avoided. A menstrual history was obtained from female participants over 11 years of age. Half the females with PWS (8/16 of the population sample) gave a history of at least one instance of spontaneous vaginal bleeding, without prior administration of sex hormones. None from the entire cohort experienced regular normal frequency of menstruation, none more than four per year, and, in general, the initial bleed occurred later than normal, (mean = 19.9 years, SD 7.0, $n = 13$), at 31 years in one case. Implications for fertility are unclear, as it is unknown whether ovulation occurs; the two known cases of people with PWS becoming pregnant have been mentioned in Chapter 2. Reports of hormone replacement, past or present, are recorded in Table 9.4.

Seizures

Results relating to seizures are reported in Table 9.5. Many of the histories were atypical but, of the seven categorised as epileptic, five were known to have received anticonvulsant medication. Most fits occurred only during childhood or adolescence with no recurrence in adult life; the *mean age of onset* was 4.7 years, with a standard deviation of 6.1. Two individuals (both adults) were currently receiving anticonvulsant medication (carbamazepine).

PWS is not characterised by seizures.[36] However, in general, the risk of seizure disorder is increased in syndromes associated with learning disability. Histories

Table 9.5. Prevalence of seizure

Condition (lifetime history)	Prevalence					
	Under 18 years		Over 17 years		All ages	
	population sample (%)	expanded cohort (%)	population sample (%)	expanded cohort (%)	population sample (%)	expanded cohort (%)
Epileptic seizure (grand mal and petit mal) ± treatment	**2/34 (6)**	4/50 (8)	**5/31 (16)**	9/56 (8)	**7/65 (11)**	13/106 (12)
Febrile convulsion (excluding above)	**4/34 (12)**	5/50 (10)	**1/31 (3)**	1/56 (1)	**5/65 (8)**	6/106 (6)
Other atypical seizures (excluding above)	**4/34 (12)**	11/50 (22)	**6/31 (19)**	13/56 (12)	**10/65 (15)**	24/106 (23)

were often atypical. At least two parents felt unable to decide whether all fits were true epileptic seizures or not, and clear distinction between febrile convulsions and seizure disorder was not always possible. Bearing in mind these reservations, our findings concurred quite closely with those of Williams *et al.*[37] in a similarly-sized study of children with PWS, although he described a higher rate of 17% having febrile convulsion, while a matched group of children with general neurodevelopmental disorder exhibited seizure rates of 23%. Of interest were the numbers of undiagnosed atypical episodes, comprising unexplained collapse, 'absences' or 'drooping'. Similar episodes were also reported in six of those who also had a more robust diagnosis of seizure. It is possible that such 'attacks' were more akin to cataplexy, which is said to be associated with PWS,[38] or other disorder of sleep regulation, though no individual had been given a definite diagnosis. It was noted that these episodes appeared more common in those individuals with maternal disomy of chromosome 15, 15/30, as compared with 10/57 of those with a deletion on the paternal chromosome.

Sleep disorders

In the population sample, 40/63 (64%) of informants reported *noisy or disturbed sleep*. Excessive daytime sleepiness was described in 47/64 (73%) of those with PWS, though in four instances this was in the past only. Thirteen (20%) had a *diagnosis of a sleep disorder*: 12 sleep apnoea, and one narcolepsy. In the expanded cohort, the mean BMI of those with a *diagnosed sleep disorder* was 36.0 kg/m^2 (sd 14.4, $n = 19$), compared with 29.6 kg/m^2 (sd 10.5, $n = 78$) in those without (significant at the level $P > 0.05$). In *reported snorers*, mean BMI was 34.1 kg/m^2 (sd 12.2,

Table 9.6. Relationship of *Epworth Daytime Sleepiness Score* to various factors, using the expanded cohort of people with Prader–Willi syndrome (PWS)

Group from expanded cohort with PWS	Mean Epworth sleepiness score	Significance using *t*-test
Those reporting disturbed/noisy sleep	8.9 (sd 5.1, $n = 63$)	
		Not significant $P > 0.05$
Those not reporting disturbed noisy sleep	8.1 (sd 4.1, $n = 33$)	
Adults 18 years and over	9.9 (sd 5.1, $n = 56$)	
		$P = 0.01$
Children under 18 years	6.9 (sd 3.6, $n = 43$)	
Those with BMI >30 kg/m^2	10.0 (sd 4.8, $n = 43$)	
		$P = 0.02$
Those with BMI <31 kg/m^2	7.5 (sd 4.5, $n = 55$)	

BMI: Body Mass Index.

$n = 65$), as opposed to 23.6 kg/m^2 (sd 6.1, $n = 31$) in *non-snorers*, but the average *age* of the *snorers* was higher: 20.6 years (sd 11.2, $n = 69$) compared with 14.6 years (sd 11.6, $n = 37$). However, only three persons with BMI greater than 30 kg/m^2 were *non-snorers*. The Epworth Daytime Sleepiness Scale[39] was used to compare different groups (see Table 9.6). *Sleep disturbance* did not appear to explain fully the *daytime sleepiness*. *Age* in itself appeared to have a significant effect, (significant at the level $P = 0.01$), as did raised BMI (significant at the level $P = 0.02$).

Sleep problems and daytime sleepiness were common, but many had not been assessed professionally for sleep disorders. Disorders of sleep may well be due to factors intrinsic to the syndrome, as well as consequent upon the obesity (see also Chapter 2). The former would include sleep disturbance secondary to hypothalamic dysfunction and structural abnormalities.[30,40] The latter would include the role of obesity as a cause of obstructive sleep apnoea. The increased daytime sleepiness scores in adulthood, as well as being linked to increased weight, may also be related to lack of activity. There were anecdotal reports that people were less sleepy if actively stimulated by tasks that they enjoyed, a more common occurrence in children.

Eye disorders

Visual problems of unspecified nature were very common, with 51/66 (77%) of the population sample reporting a *visual problem* of some kind. Apart from *strabismus* (see Table 9.2), the nature of the visual defect was not always identified. The

Table 9.7. Other relevant findings in the population group

Condition (lifetime history)	Prevalence in population sample (%)		
	Under 18 years	Over 17 years	All ages
Frequent constipation	5/34 (15)	8/32 (25)	13/66 (20)
Frequent diarrhoea	11/34 (32)	6/32 (19)	17/66 (26)
History of ENT surgery			13/63 (21)
History of hernia			4/66 (6)
Club foot/foot deformity			5/66 (8)
Congenital hip problems			5/66 (6)

ENT: ear, nose and throat.

prevalence of *visual problems* was similar to reported rates in children with Down syndrome who themselves are five times more likely to wear glasses than the general population.[41] However, the rate of *strabismus* (Table 9.2), though comparable to that identified in previous PWS studies,[42,43] was greater than that found in other learning disabled groups, such as those with Down syndrome, where about 27% report the condition and 9% undergo surgical correction.[41,44] In the present study, the defect had not always been confirmed by ophthalmic testing and the particular facial appearance of people with PWS can give an erroneous impression. Strabismus has been linked to hypopigmentation associated with misrouting of optic fibres,[43] but no correlation was found in this group between those with the disorder and those who were fair in relation to their family background. High levels of refractive errors have been implicated. We were unable to test this, as informants were often unsure about the nature of other ophthalmic defects. General neuromotor dysfunction, as signified by the hypotonia, has also been proposed as an explanation for the high prevalence of strabismus.[42] People with PWS are reported to be susceptible to a variety of ophthalmic problems[42] and these observations underline the care needed when assessing visual function.

Other findings

Other relevant health problems in the population group are shown in Table 9.7. There was evidence that many people with PWS had difficulties appreciating pain and temperature (see also Chapter 2), and exhibiting other common symptoms of illness. Fifty (76%) of the population group were considered to have a *raised pain threshold*, confirmed in 33 by descriptions of clearly inappropriate responses to trauma. Thirty-seven (56%) were thought to have difficulty appreciating temperature; many required bath and shower temperatures to be pre-set or monitored. Vomiting was unknown or extremely rare in 85% individuals ($n = 55$).

Constipation and/or diarrhoea were common minor problems. Levels of constipation in children were similar to those reported in children with Down syndrome[41] and may be related to lack of muscle tone, or the strict dietary regimen necessary for an individual with PWS. Anecdotally, there were also problems reported in maintaining fluid intake. Diarrhoea was more common in children and attributed to dietary indiscretion or to gastro-intestinal infection, occurring in place of vomiting.

Results from questions pertaining to general medical history revealed little other significant pathology. Levels of routine ear, nose and throat surgery were low, despite possible concern about obstructive apnoea. Of interest were those conditions possibly associated with hypotonia and muscle weakness (Table 9.7). In addition to the specific conditions noted, 13/108 participants volunteered information relating to general joint laxity and frequent sprains or dislocations. In view of the obesity, one might have expected a high prevalence of arthritis. However, only two people with such problems were reported in the entire cohort, the knees being affected in both. It may be that joints are not subject to stress because of the low levels of activity.

Discussion

The study is population-based and therefore the findings are unlikely to be distorted by significant selection effects. Although all participants, their main carers and others were interviewed, physical examinations were not undertaken. Self-reporting and information from main carers were the only sources of information. Thus, for disorders such as scoliosis and hypertension, the findings are likely to be an underestimate. Furthermore, in the absence of clinical investigations, the presence or not of pre-diabetic states could not be ascertained. An interesting observation is that other illnesses, although inquired about, were relatively rare. Anecdotally, parents often described their offspring as suffering fewer illnesses than other members of the family. It could be postulated that features of PWS (i.e. decreased perception of pain and temperature, inactive lifestyle, decreased propensity to vomit) may hide early symptoms, so underlying pathologies remain undetected. In addition, an illness may not become apparent until a fairly advanced stage, when recovery may be compromised by the stress imposed on the cardio-pulmonary system by long-term obesity. This is supported by reports of individuals who do not necessarily experience frequent illness but who quickly become seriously ill. Two participants, both with BMI greater than 60 kg/m^2, suffered serious illness of sudden onset, one of a cardio-pulmonary nature, prior to the study period. Given estimates of the mortality rate in this population (see Chapter 4) and the fact that no one older than 46 years was positively identified, the level of overt life-threatening morbidity during the lifetime of the participants seemed surprisingly low. It is possible that those with more severe health problems may have been included in the group of non-responders. On the other hand, relatively fit individuals, especially adults, may never have been suspected of having PWS. Among the potential cohort, one death of unknown cause was reported during the ascertainment period.

Whilst the risk of disorders such as strabismus and scoliosis may relate to core features of the syndrome (e.g. hypotonia), this may not be so for NIDDM or hypertension. We propose that these are likely to be secondary to the severe obesity that can develop and that they are therefore preventable. Although obesity was originally considered a central feature of the syndrome, our current understanding points to a failure of satiation and resultant over-eating as being the crucial abnormality. Thus, managing the food environment and controlling access to food is the key issue.[45]

We conclude that those with PWS have the potential for developing serious specific health problems in childhood and in later life. Some of these are preventable with good management of the person's diet, hormone replacement therapy and by regular health surveillance. Others may not be readily preventable but indicate the need for health surveillance and, if necessary, appropriate intervention.

REFERENCES

1. Laurance, B., Brito, A. & Wilkinson, J. Prader–Willi syndrome after age 15 years. *Archives of Disease in Childhood* **56** (1981), 181–186.
2. Butler, M. G. Prader–Willi syndrome: current understanding of cause and diagnosis. *American Journal of Medical Genetics* **35** (1990), 319–332.
3. Prader, A., Labhart, A. & Willi, H. Ein Syndrom von Adipositas, Kleinwuchs, Kryptorchismus und Oligophrenie nach myatonieartigem Zustandim Neugeborenenalter. *Schweizerische Medizinische Wochenschrift* **86** (1956), 1260–1261.
4. Lamb, A. S. & Johnson, W. M. Premature coronary artery atherosclerosis in a patient with Prader–Willi syndrome. *American Journal of Medical Genetics* **28** (1987), 873–880.
5. Holm, V. A., Cassidy, S. B., Butler, M. G. *et al.* Prader–Willi syndrome: consensus diagnostic criteria. *Pediatrics* **91** (1993), 398–402.
6. Hákonarson, H., Moskovitz, J., Daigle, K., Cassidy, S. & Cloutier, M. Pulmonary function abnormalities in Prader–Willi syndrome. *Journal of Pediatrics* **126** (1995), 565–569.
7. Alexander, R. C., Van Dyke, D. C. & Hanson, J. W. Overview. In Greenswag, L. R. & Alexander, R. C. (Eds). *Management of Prader–Willi syndrome*, 2nd edn. pp. 3–17. New York: Springer-Verlag, 1995.
8. Cox, B. D., Blaxter, M., Buckle, A. L. J. *et al.* The Health and Lifestyle Survey. London: Health Promotion Research Trust, 1987.

9. Schuster, D. P., Osei, K. & Zipf, W. B. Characterization of alterations in glucose and insulin metabolism in Prader–Willi subjects. *Metabolism* **45** (1996), 1514–1520.

10. Vanderpump, P. J., Tunbridge, W. M. G., French, J. M. *et al.* The incidence of diabetes mellitus in an English community: a 20-year follow-up of the Whickham survey. *Diabetic Medicine* **13** (1996), 741–747.

11. Rabkin, S. W., Chen, Y., Leiter, L., Liu, L. & Reeder, B. A. Risk factor correlates of body mass index. *Canadian Medical Association Journal* **157** (Suppl. 1) (1997), 526–531.

12. Must, A., Spadano, J., Coakley, E. H., Field, A. E., Colditz, G. & Dietz, W. H. The disease burden associated with overweight and obesity. *Journal of the American Medical Association* **282** (1999), 1523–1529.

13. Bray, G. A. Obesity increases risk for diabetes. *International Journal of Obesity* **16** (Suppl. 4) (1992), s13–17.

14. Goya Wannamethee, S. & Shaper, A. G. Weight change and duration of overweight and obesity in the incidence of Type 2 diabetes. *Diabetes Care* **22** (1999), 1266–1272.

15. Pinhas-Hamiel, O., Dolan, L. M., Daniels, S. R., Standiford, D., Khoury, P. R. & Zeitler, P. Increased incidence of non-insulin-dependent diabetes mellitus among adolescents. *Journal of Pediatrics* **128** (1996), 608–615.

16. Davies, P. S. W. & Joughin, C. Using stable isotopes to assess reduced physical activity of individuals with Prader–Willi syndrome. *American Journal of Mental Retardation* **98** (1993), 349–353.

17. Hu, F. B., Sigal, R. J., Rich-Edwards, J. W. *et al.* Walking compared with vigorous physical activity and risk of Type 2 diabetes in women. *Journal of the American Medical Association* **282** (1999), 1433–1439.

18. Ashwell, M. Obesity in men and women. *International Journal of Obesity* **18** (1994), S1–S7.

19. Greenswag, L. R. Adults with Prader–Willi syndrome: a survey of 232 cases. *Developmental Medicine & Child Neurology* **29** (1987), 145–152.

20. Anderson, R., Britton, J., Esmail, A., Hollowell, J. & Strachan, D. Respiratory disease and Sudden Infant Death syndrome. In Botting B. (Ed.). *The Health of our Children: Decennial Supplement: the Registrar General's Decennial Supplement for England and Wales*, pp. 113–125. London: HMSO, 1995.

21. Brooks, H. L., Azen, S. P., Gerberg, E., Brooks, R. & Chan, L. Scoliosis: a prospective epidemiological study. *Journal of Bone and Joint Surgery (American)* **57A** (1975), 968–972.

22. Holm, V. A. & Laurnen, E. L. Prader–Willi syndrome and scoliosis. *Developmental Medicine and Child Neurology* **23** (1981), 192–201.

23. Gurd, A. R. & Thompson, T. R. Scoliosis in Prader–Willi syndrome. *Journal of Pediatric Orthopedics* **1** (1981), 317–320.

24. Rees, D., Jones, M. W., Owen, R. & Dorgan, J. C. Scoliosis surgery in the Prader–Willi syndrome. *Journal of Bone and Joint Surgery (Britain)* **71** (1989), 685–687.

25. Cassidy, S. B., Rubin, K. G. & Mukaida, C. S. Osteoporosis in Prader–Willi syndrome. *American Journal of Human Genetics* **37** (1985), A49.

26. Herman, R., Mixon, J., Fisher, A., Maulucci, R. & Stuyck, J. Idiopathic scoliosis and the central nervous system: a motor control problem. *Spine* **10** (1985), 1–14.

27. Soriano, R. M. G., Weisz, I. & Houghton, G. R. Scoliosis in the Prader–Willi syndrome. *Spine* **13** (1988), 209–211.

28. Brambilla, P., Bosio, L., Manzoni, P., Pietrobelli, A., Beccaria, L. & Chiumello, G. Peculiar body composition in patients with Prader–Labhart–Willi syndrome. *American Journal of Clinical Nutrition* **65** (1997), 1369–1374.

29. Driscoll, D. J., Smith, B. M., Silverstein, J. H., Rosenbloom, A. L., Theriaque, D. W. & Hutson, A. Medical issues in adults with Prader–Willi syndrome. Paper presented at the *4th triennial IPWSO Scientific Conference 2001, Saint Paul, Minnesota, USA.*

30. Swaab, D. F. Prader–Willi syndrome and the hypothalamus. *Acta Paediatrica Supplement* **423** (1997), 50–54.

31. Lee, P. D. K. Endocrine and metabolic aspects of Prader–Willi syndrome. In Greenswag, L. R. & Alexander, R. C. (Eds). *Management of Prader–Willi Syndrome*, 2nd edn., pp. 32–57. New York: Springer-Verlag, 1995.

32. O'Halloran, D. J., Tstsoulis, A., Whitehouse, R. W., Holmes, S. J., Adams, J. E. & Shalet, S. M. Increased bone density after recombinant human growth hormone (GH) therapy in adults with isolated GH deficiency. *Journal of Clinical Endocrinology and Metabolism* **76** (1993), 1344–1348.

33. Davies, P. S. W., Evans, S., Broomhead, S. *et al.* Effect of growth hormone on height, weight, and body composition in Prader–Willi syndrome. *Archives of Disease in Childhood* **78** (1998), 174–176.

34. Lindgren, A. C., Hagenäs, L., Müller, J. *et al.* Growth hormone treatment of children with Prader–Willi syndrome affects linear growth and body composition favourably. *Acta Paediatrica* **87** (1998), 28–31.

35. Carrel, A. L., Myers, S. E., Whitman, B. Y. & Allen, D. B. Growth hormone improves body composition, fat utilisation, physical strength and agility, and growth in Prader–Willi syndrome: a controlled study. *Journal of Pediatrics* **134** (1999), 215–221.

36. Cassidy, S. B. & Schwartz, S. Prader–Willi and Angelman syndromes disorders of genomic imprinting. *Medicine* **77** (1998), 40–151.

37. Williams, M. S., Rooney, B. L., Williams, J., Josephson, K. & Pauli, R. Investigation of thermoregulatory characteristics in patients with Prader–Willi syndrome. *American Journal of Medical Genetics* **49** (1994), 302–307.

38. Helbing-Zwanenburg, B., Kamphuisen, H. A. & Mourtazaev, M. S. The origin of excessive daytime sleepiness in the Prader–Willi syndrome. *Journal of Intellectual Disability Research* **37** (1993), 533–541.

39. Johns, M. W. A new method for measuring daytime sleepiness: the Epworth Sleepiness Scale. *Sleep* **14** (1991), 540–545.

40. Clift, S., Dahlitz, M. & Parkes, J. D. Sleep apnoea in the Prader–Willi syndrome. *Journal of Sleep Research* **3** (1994), 121–126.

41. Leonard, S., Bower, C., Petteson, B. & Leonard, H. Medical aspects of school-aged children with Down syndrome. *Developmental Medicine and Child Neurology* **41** (1999), 683–688.

42. Hered, R. W., Rogers, S., Zang, Y.-F. & Biglan, A. W. Ophthalmologic features of Prader–Willi syndrome. *Journal of Pediatric Ophthalmology and Strabismus* **25** (1988), 145–150.

43. Creel, D. J., Bendel, C. M., Wiesner, G. L., Wirtschafter, J. D., Arthur, D. C. & King, R. A. Abnormalities of the central visual pathways in Prader–Willi syndrome associated with hypopigmentation. *New England Journal of Medicine* **314** (1986), 1606–1609.

44. Turner, S., Sloper, P., Cunningham, C. & Knussen, C. Health problems in children with Down's syndrome. *Child: Care, Health and Development* **16** (1990), 83–97.

45. Holland, A. J. Understanding the eating disorder affecting people with Prader–Willi syndrome. *Journal of Applied Research in Intellectual Disorders* **11** (1998), 192–206.

10

Psychiatric illness

Prevalence of psychiatric illness in people with learning disabilities (LD) may be slightly higher than that in the normal population, especially when the difficulties of diagnosis in the learning disabled population is taken into account. Cooper & Collacott,[1] in a review article, suggested that rates of affective disorder among people with a learning disability may be as low as 1–5%. Corbett,[2] in his Camberwell study of people with LD, aged 15 years and older, found rates of present or past significant affective disorders of 5.5%. A population-based study of adults with Down syndrome reported rates of depression of 11%.[3] Psychiatrists working with people with PWS have come to speculate that rates in PWS may be higher than those in the general LD population, and that general depression and anxiety may not be the most common symptoms found in PWS. A study that looked at psychiatric symptoms in 23 people with PWS (genetically confirmed in 20 cases) and a comparison group of 73 people with other LD[4] found higher rates of affective disorder (4/23 v. 3/73), schizophrenia/delusional disorder (1/23 v. 2/73), and obsessive–compulsive disorder (OCD) (1/23 v. 2/73) in PWS compared with other causes for LD. Unlike the LD group, there were no cases of generalised anxiety disorder, agoraphobia, other phobias, alcoholism, dementia or autism in the PWS group. In a group of 35 adolescents with PWS,[5] it was estimated that more than half had definite or probable DSM-III[6] diagnoses, compared with 18.7% of the general population. Diagnoses were predominantly of neurotic disorders, but suspiciousness, 'strange' ideation and auditory or visual hallucinations were also reported. Twelve of the 35 had occasional auditory hallucinations.

In the last decade two disorders in particular have come to be linked more specifically with PWS: psychosis and OCD. In the study by Beardsmore *et al.*[4] described above, the four people with PWS who were considered to have an affective disorder all showed psychotic symptoms, and OCD was slightly more prevalent in the PWS group (although by only a single person). This chapter is concerned with our Cambridge group's research into the prevalence of affective psychosis in PWS, while Chapter 11 explores obsessive–compulsive symptoms.

Most of the reports of psychotic symptoms in PWS are single case studies, particularly the earlier ones, and generally they detail onset, symptoms, medication, response to medication, remission and follow-up. We need to bear in mind that, in the early reports, the diagnosis of PWS was based only on clinical criteria and so we cannot be certain that the people in the reports had the PWS genotype. This is important in the light of the Cambridge study findings. One of the earliest reports of psychotic symptoms in PWS was that of Kollrack & Wolff in 1966.[7] They described a 20-year-old man with clinically diagnosed PWS who suffered two brief psychotic episodes. Other single case studies were published between 1987 and 1993.[8,9,10,11] Two further case studies were reported in 1997,[12,13] both concerned females in their late teens (19 and 17 years of age) with PWS of maternal disomy genetic subtype. Both showed extreme anxiety and psychotic symptoms. These people have in common a rapid onset of illness with no readily apparent trigger and a fairly rapid response to antipsychotic medication. Recurrence rates varied from nil to regular episodes, although this may depend on whether or not medication was continued in some form.

The prevalence of psychotic symptoms in people with PWS has been estimated in various ways. Bray et al.[14] described assessment of a series of 40 people with PWS, of whom two had symptoms described as hallucinations and withdrawal, and both required admission. Whitman & Accardo[5] looked at symptoms in 35 adolescents with PWS and found 12 with occasional auditory hallucinations. Bartolucci & Younger[15] reported that four out of nine people with PWS had additional psychotic symptoms. Two studies in 1998,[4,16] based respectively on 23 and 95 people with PWS, found 26% with lifetime psychotic symptoms and 6.3% with one month prevalence of psychotic symptoms, respectively.

Although those with PWS have differed somewhat in symptomatology, many have in common the characteristics described above: sudden onset with no clear trigger and rapid response to antipsychotic medication. Persecutory delusions, agitation, anxiety and disturbed sleep have been almost universally reported and many people have shown a cyclical affective disorder. Diagnoses have ranged from schizophrenia to bipolar affective disorder to cycloid psychosis.

In most of the early studies referenced above, PWS has been diagnosed clinically. The later prevalence studies did attempt genetic confirmation of PWS, but none achieved 100% genetic diagnoses. Genetic subtypes of PWS were not commonly specified prior to the early 1990s. The case studies of Wanatabe et al.[12] and Whittaker et al.[13] were people with PWS both with maternal disomies. The reports by Clarke et al.,[17] Verhoeven et al.,[18] and Beardsmore et al.[4] included five, four and three cases of people with PWS respectively in which genetic subtypes were known.

These subtypes comprised, respectively: three deletion, one disomy and one other; one deletion, three disomy; and one deletion and two disomy (erroneously reported as two deletion, one disomy in the reference).

In order to test the hypothesis that there is a specific link between PWS and the risk of affective disorders and/or other psychotic illnesses, we determined the prevalence of these disorders in a population-based sample of people with PWS. In addition, we investigated whether the presence of either chromosomal 15 disomies or deletions were specifically associated with any increase that might have been observed.

Our study of psychiatric illness in PWS was based on the 65 (34 children, 31 adults) people in the population sample who were considered to meet clinical and/or genetic criteria for PWS. In the case of 29 children and 26 adults, the exact type of genetic abnormality was established, either from previous health records or, if consent had been given for venepuncture, from molecular and cytogenetic analysis. As none of those below the age of 18 years screened positively (see below) for possible psychotic or affective disorders, it was the 26 adults, in whom the genetic diagnosis of PWS had been confirmed, that made up the cohort for this study.

As detailed in Chapters 3 and 4, all those referred from different sources as possibly having PWS were assessed by a chartered psychologist and a medically qualified research assistant. Information was obtained from the person with PWS and from a family member or paid carer. On the basis of this information and the behaviour of the person with PWS during the researchers' visit, the researchers applied a screen as to whether or not the person should be seen by a psychiatrist specialising in the assessment of people with LD. Those with clinically and/or genetically confirmed PWS and a definite, or suspected, history of mental illness, or for whom the informant indicated more than transitory episodes of severe depression or anxiety or other nervous state, or who were receiving, or had been prescribed, psychotropic medication, or whose behaviour or personality had undergone a major change, or whose behaviour during the visit gave rise to suspicion in the minds of the researchers, screened positive. As with the original ascertainment of people with PWS, the screen was intentionally over-inclusive. The assessing psychiatrist made the diagnosis based on ICD-10 criteria[19] and, using case vignettes, this was also undertaken independently by two further psychiatrists, blind to any knowledge of the others' diagnoses or the participants' chromosomal status. As all those confirmed to have had a psychotic disorder were over the age of 28 years when seen by the researchers, all others at that age or above were also seen, to ensure that the screening technique had not missed any with an affective or psychotic disorder. The psychiatric assessments included interviews with the participant and main carer, and a review of general practitioner and psychiatric notes, with the participant's consent. The presence and nature of any psychiatric illness in the past or at present was thereby established.

None aged under 18 years and 10 of the 26 (38%) aged 18 years or older scored positively on screening as possibly having a psychotic illness and/or an affective disorder. At full psychiatric assessment, and with 100% consensus between the three psychiatrists who reviewed the evidence, six of these ten candidates were finally considered to have had such an illness. The *psychiatric diagnoses, age of the participant, approximate age of onset of psychiatric disorder, IQ, Body Mass Index (BMI) at the time seen, chromosomal status* and *psychiatric symptomatology* are given in Table 10.1. There were six other people with PWS over the age of 28 in the population sample. Five of these six participants over the age of 28 consented to be assessed by a psychiatrist, and their details are also included in Table 10.1 (participants 11 to 15). One of the five was assessed positively, again by all three psychiatrists. This woman had initially been screened as having autism.

Of the 15 participants, seen for detailed psychiatric assessments, three were diagnosed as having no psychiatric disorder, one was diagnosed as having a behaviour disorder; the remaining 11 had, or had had, a psychiatric disorder, predominately affective in nature. All three psychiatrists independently agreed that seven of the 11 (cases 1, 2, 4, 6, 7, 9 and 11) met criteria for a major affective or psychotic disorder. The prevalence rate of severe psychiatric disorder in the 26 adults was therefore 27%.

Chromosome type

Table 10.2 lists the presence or absence of a severe affective or psychotic disorder in different age groups and the chromosome types. Of the 26 adults of known genetic status in this study, 13 (50%) had a chromosome 15 deletion, eight (31%) uniparental disomy and one (4%) an imprinting centre mutation. Three others had the characteristic methylation pattern diagnostic of PWS and were found to have small chromosomal deletions. Of the seven with a psychotic illness, one had a deletion, one an imprinting error, and the remaining five (71%) all had uniparental heterodisomies. All the participants with uniparental disomies, 28 years or over in age, had had a psychotic illness. When the deletion and disomy groups were compared for rates of psychotic illness, there was a significant ($P < 0.05$) risk ratio of 8.125 (95% confidence interval (CI) 1.15;57.6) between the two, as there was for those aged 28 years or older with a risk ratio of 9.0 (95% CI 1.42;57.1) between deletion and disomy groups.

Table 10.1. ICD-10 diagnoses for 15 people with Prader–Willi syndrome

Case	Gender	Clinical diagnosis	Age (years)	Medication	Age of onset (years)	IQ	BMI (kg/m^2)	Genetic abnormality	Psychotic symptoms
1	F	Depressive psychosis	47	a,b,c	21	71	31	Del15q11–q13	Paranoid delusions
2	M	Bipolar affective disorder	29	a,b,c	19	65	37	Imprinting mutation	None
3	F	Depressive episode	33	c	32	78	74	Del15q11–q13	None
4	M	Psychotic disorder	41	a,b,c	28	62	43	Maternal heterodisomy	Paranoid delusions and hallucinations
5	M	Behavioural problems	33	a,b		53	24	Del15q11–q13	None
6	F	Bipolar affective disorder	46	a	29	59	34	Maternal heterodisomy	Paranoid delusions and hallucinations
7	F	Depressive psychosis	39	c	22	70	29	Maternal heterodisomy	Paranoid delusions and hallucinations
8	M	Mild depressive episode	39	c	36	91	32	Del15q11–q13	None
9	F	Psychotic disorder	38	a,b,c	36	73	29	Maternal heterodisomy	Paranoid delusions and hallucinations
10	M	Past depressive episode	36			68	52	Del15q11–q13	None
11	F	Bipolar affective disorder	34	c	29	48	26	Maternal heterodisomy	Paranoid delusions and hallucinations
12	M	None	39			51	?	Del15q11–q13	None
13	F	None	37			62	48	Del15q11–q13	None
14	M	Mild depressive episode	47	a,c	47	61	42	Del15q11–q13	None
15	M	None	40			68	31	Del15q11–q13	None

a: antipsychotic; b: mood stabiliser; c: antidepressant.

BMI: Body Mass Index.

Case 2 paternal contribution at D15S11, D15S210 and D15S97, but not at D15S128.

Cases 12, 13 and 14 heterozygous at D15S165.

Table 10.2. Numbers of people with Prader–Willi syndrome with psychotic disorders in relation to age (years) and genetic disorder. Total numbers within brackets

	Age 18–27	Age 28+
Deletion (15q11–q13)	0 (4)	1 (9)
Uniparental disomy	0 (3)	5 (5)
Other	0 (3)	1 (1)
Total	0 (10)	7 (15)

Risk of psychotic illness

If a lifetime risk of severe psychotic illness in the learning disabled population is considered to be 3%, then the chance that five people with PWS due to chromosome 15 disomy, drawn at random from an older adult age group, would all have experienced such a disorder by chance, would be of the order of $(3/100)$.[5] Even if the baseline rate for psychotic illness is taken to be that found in the older deletion group (10%), the probability that all five would have developed psychotic illness by chance is still remote $(1/10^5)$. It therefore seems unlikely that these findings would have arisen by chance, or that the risk of developing a psychotic illness is due to having PWS. Rather, it would appear to be very particularly related to the presence of two copies of the maternal chromosome 15. This might also account for the presence of psychotic illness in the one person with an imprinting centre mutation, as a failure to reset the normal gender specific imprinting pattern could give rise to the equivalent of a maternal disomy over that part of chromosome 15.

This study represents the first epidemiological study of psychotic illnesses in adults with PWS. The strength of this study is its population base that allows an estimate of the prevalence of such psychiatric disorders affecting people with PWS to be ascertained free from potential selection bias. Establishing the exact psychiatric diagnosis can be problematic in people with additional LD. However, there was high agreement that cyclical affective disorders with psychotic phenomenology were the main characteristics of the seven diagnosed as having a major psychiatric illness. The one person of the seven with a chromosome 15 deletion had a less obviously affective disorder. She had previously been reported[17] (case 2 of reference 16) and she has been treated with trifluoperazine for many years.

For the purpose of comparison, we have considered published studies of the prevalence rates of psychiatric disorder among people with LD generally, and those of specific disorders associated with learning disabilities.[1,2,3] The high prevalence rate for severe psychiatric illness in people with PWS is therefore unlikely to

Table 10.3. Recent articles describing people with Prader–Willi syndrome and major psychiatric disorder

Reference (listing)	Number in study	Genetics known	Genetic abnormality			Comments
			Del	Dis	Other	
Clarke, 1998 (16)	6	5	3	1	1	Includes participant 1 in this study
Verhoeven et al., 1998 (18)	6	4	1	3	0	
Beardsmore et al., 1998 (4)	5	3	2 (1)	1 (2)	0	Includes participants 6 and 9 in this study[a]
Wanatabe et al., 1997 (12)	1	1	0	1	0	Recurrent brief depression with psychotic symptoms
Whittaker et al., 1997 (13)	1	1	0	1	0	Psychotic illness
Takhar, 1997 (37)	1	0[b]	0	0	0	Schizophrenic psychosis
Vogels et al., 2003 (20)	6	6	0	5	1	Other = imprinting centre defect. All had experienced a psychotic episode

Del: deletion; Dis: disomy.

[a] In the paper by Beardsmore participant No 9 of our study was incorrectly reported as having a deletion when in fact a maternal disomy 15 was present. The corrected number in each chromosome group is given in parentheses.

[b] metaphase banding failed to locate any chromosome abnormality.

be due to having a learning disability, but would appear to represent an increased risk specific to this syndrome. However, our findings of the relationship between psychosis and the chromosomal type of PWS would suggest that it is not the syndrome per se that is associated with this very high risk of psychotic illness, but rather a combination of age and the presence of maternal chromosome 15 disomy. Strikingly, five of the seven (71%) of those with severe affective and/or psychotic disorders had maternal uniparental heterodisomy. There was no one with PWS due to maternal chromosome 15 disomy aged 28 years or older who had not had a psychotic illness, suggesting that it is this chromosomal abnormality that is particularly associated with the high risk for severe psychiatric disorder.

The numbers in this study are small and further study is required to determine whether the presence of maternal chromosome 15 disomies are inevitably associated with development of affective and psychotic symptomatology in later life. However, there is some support for this observation from case reports where those with chromosome 15 disomies were more common than would be expected. In Table 10.3 we have summarised the results of recent articles and case reports. For example, Verhoeven et al.[18] reported six people with PWS and an affective disorder or cycloid psychosis. Three of the four with known genetics had uniparental disomy. A subsequent report of similar findings from the Belgian longitudinal study of PWS[20] supports our observation of an elevated prevalence of psychotic disorder in the disomy subtype of PWS.

If this observation of the relationship between the rarer genetic form of PWS and severe psychiatric illness were to be confirmed by further studies, it would have significant implications, both for people with PWS and for our understanding of the possible genetic basis of such psychiatric disorders and the chromosomal site for a putative candidate gene for psychotic disorder. Given this difference in rates of psychotic illness between the two chromosomal types of PWS, we hypothesise that the increased risk of severe psychiatric disorder in those with the disomy form of PWS may be due to different patterns of gene expression between these two chromosomal types. Whilst there would be no predicted difference between those with PWS due to chromosome 15 deletions and chromosome 15 disomy in the expression of maternally imprinted genes located within the PWS critical region (PWSCR), there would be for those maternally imprinted genes outside the PWSCR, and paternally imprinted genes both inside and outside the PWSCR (see Table 6.1). Thus, in the case of maternally imprinted genes outside the PWSCR, neither allele would be expressed in those with maternal disomy, but one would be in those with deletions. For any paternally imprinted genes located inside or outside the PWSCR, both alleles would be expressed in those with maternal disomy, rather than the normal one. As all with disomy were heterodisomies, this also excludes the possibility that an autosomal recessive gene predisposing to psychotic illness has been uncovered.

A further observation is that the affective and psychotic illnesses all started in adult life. This is consistent with the understanding of psychotic illness as a predominately adult disorder. However, it raises the hypothesis that imprinted gene(s) on chromosome 15 may be normally switched on or off in early adult life. Thus, if further investigation was to confirm our present observation, it provides a strong case for a candidate gene for major affective disorder on chromosome 15. A search for imprinted genes and investigation of mRNA expression, comparing expression patterns of adults with different chromosomal types of PWS, would therefore be of considerable interest. This has now been done for the PWS region (see Chapter 8).

We can also ask if these findings for people with PWS have any relevance to the general population. Can similar gene expression differences occur through other mechanisms in the general population, and if so, would they result in the development of a psychotic illness? It is well established that in the major mental illnesses and in many other psychiatric disorders there is evidence of genetic vulnerability. In addition, genetic influences also underpin many behavioural/personality traits that may have been shaped over time through selection pressures. With respect to candidate genes, the possible links to chromosome 15 have included panic disorder,[21,22] bipolar disorder[23,24,25] and schizophrenia.[26,27,28,29] In panic disorder, an interstitial duplication 15q24–q26, is known to be involved. In bipolar disorder and schizophrenia, linkage studies have implicated regions of chromosome 15; with *GABRA5*, the *GABA-A* receptor alpha5 subunit, as a possible candidate for bipolar disorder and *CHRNA7*, the alpha7 neuronal nicotinic acetylcholine receptor subunit, a possible candidate for schizophrenia. The link with bipolar disorder needs further investigation, in particular, whether the link is due to those cases with psychotic symptoms. It is of note that GABA as a transmitter has been implicated in affective disorders possibly through its action on 5-HT function, adding support to this receptor gene being a candidate gene.[30]

The model we propose to account for the increasing age-related rates of psychotic illness in those with PWS due to chromosome 15 disomy would indicate that the propensity to psychotic illness is dependent on 100% increase of the gene product (if the gene is paternally imprinted) or absence of expression (if the gene is maternally imprinted). We propose three possible genetic models that might lead to actual or functional gene dosage differences in the general population and in turn to an increased vulnerability to psychotic illness. First, if this gene is imprinted, variations of the one active allele may have a more critical phenotypic effect and there may be a variant in the population that increases the propensity to psychotic illness. Second, there may be an interstitial deletion of this gene. If the chromosome 15 interstitial deletion was inherited from a parent, the gender of which would normally have resulted in that gene being imprinted, then it would have no phenotypic effect, but if inherited via the parent of the other gender where it would normally be expressed, there would be complete absence of expression of that gene (the other allele being imprinted). A similar scenario exists for the third option, that of a gene duplication. If this were inherited on the chromosome from the gender that would normally result in expression of that particular gene, there would be a double dose of gene expression due to the duplication. However, if on the chromosome from the other parent, it would be imprinted and have no phenotypic effect.

A report of a partial trisomy (including the PWS region) of chromosome 15 in a female diagnosed with bipolar disorder[31] suggests that over-expression may be responsible. If this were the mechanism, the gene would have to be paternally imprinted, and inherited on the chromosome 15 of maternal origin to result in psychotic illness. A duplication of a small part of chromosome 15 would be similar to that associated with panic disorder[21,22] and to some cases of autism[32] and would be likely to occur in the unstable PWS region, associated by linkage studies with bipolar disorder. Any of these models would be supported by the observation of inheritance patterns that might skip generations depending on the gender of the parent of origin of that gene. Risk would be dependent on the gender of the parent from which the putative gene was inherited.

Ewald *et al.*[23] found no evidence of a linkage between two $GABA_A$ subtype markers in the 15q11–q12 region and manic-depressive illness, and commented that the fact that psychosis is not an obligate feature of PWS may be explained if a gene involved in the aetiology of psychosis is located at one of the borders of the 15q11–q13 region. A recent chromosome workshop[33] indicated that 15q13–q15 is a promising region for the phenotype for functional psychosis.

Indirect evidence of possibly similar underlying brain mechanisms come from recent research on deep white matter lesions in bipolar disorder, revealed by magnetic resonance imaging scans.[34] Although such lesions are fairly common in old age, they are more common at all ages in people with bipolar disorder, especially in younger age groups.[34,35] Whether or not such lesions are related to the poor memory and attention deficits observed in those with bipolar disorder or in old age remains to be seen. However, in bipolar disorder with psychosis they are associated with a diminution of cognitive speed. In the population-based survey of PWS (all ages), cognitive differences were observed between the genetic subtypes: disomies having higher average verbal IQ, but lower performance IQ. Importantly two subtests were significantly different between the two PWS genetic subtypes: those with PWS due to disomies had higher average Vocabulary (word definitions) scores, but lower Coding (cognitive speed) scores.[36] This slower cognitive speed is similar to that found in those with bipolar disorder and white matter lesions.

Further research regarding the genetics of the non-deletion area of chromosome 15 (including the effect of imprinting) may be of benefit, not only for people with PWS, but to improve our understanding of the genetics of psychotic disorders in general. Our findings would suggest that the presence of chromosome 15 maternal disomy inevitably leads to a severe psychotic illness in early adult life. If this is correct we believe it is the only example of such a strong association between a genetic abnormality and affective psychotic illness so far reported.

REFERENCES

1. Cooper, S.-A. & Collacott, R. A. Depressive episodes in adults with learning disabilities. *Irish Journal of Psychological Medicine* **13** (1996), 105–113.
2. Corbett, J. A. Psychiatric morbidity and mental retardation. In James, F. E. & Snaith, R. P. (Eds). *Psychiatric Illness and Mental Handicap*, pp. 11–25. London: Gaskell, 1979.
3. Collacott, R. A., Cooper, S.-A. & McGrother, C. Differential rates of psychiatric disorders in adults with Down's syndrome compared with other mentally handicapped adults. *British Journal of Psychiatry* **161** (1992), 671–674.

4. Beardsmore, A., Dorman, T., Cooper, S.-A. & Webb, T. Affective psychosis and Prader–Willi syndrome. *Journal of Intellectual Disability Research* **42** (1998), 463–471.

5. Whitman, B. Y. & Accardo, P. J. Emotional symptoms in Prader–Willi syndrome adolescents. *American Journal of Medical Genetics* **28** (1987), 897–905.

6. American Psychiatric Association. *Diagnostic and Statistical Manual of Mental Disorders*, 3rd edn. Washington, DC: American Psychiatric Association, 1980.

7. Kollrack, H. W. & Wolff, D. Paranoid-halluzinatorische Psychose bei Prader–Labhart–Willi–Fanconi syndrome. *Acta Paedopsychiatrica* **33** (1966), 309–314.

8. Gupta, B. K., Fish, D. N. & Yerevanian, B. I. Carbamazepine for intermittent explosive disorder in a Prader–Willi syndrome patient. *Journal of Clinical Psychiatry* **48** (1987), 423.

9. Bhate, M. S., Robertson, P. E., Davison, E. V. & Brummit, J. H. Prader–Willi syndrome with hypothyroidism. *Journal of Mental Deficiency Research* **33** (1989), 235–244.

10. Tu, J.-B., Hartridge, C. & Izawa, J. Psychopharmacogenetic aspects of Prader–Willi syndrome. *Journal of the American Academy of Child and Adolescent Psychiatry* **31** (1992), 1137–1140.

11. Jerome, L. Prader–Willi syndrome and bipolar illness. *Journal of the American Academy of Child and Adolescent Psychiatry* **32** (1993), 876–877.

12. Watanabe, H., Ohmori, O. & Abe, K. Recurrent brief depression in Prader–Willi syndrome: a case report. *Psychiatric Genetics* **7** (1997), 41–44.

13. Whittaker, J. F., Cooper, C., Harrington, R. C. & Price, D. A. Prader–Willi syndrome and acute psychosis. *International Journal of Psychiatry in Clinical Practice* **1** (1997), 217–219.

14. Bray, G. A., Dahms, W. T., Swerdloff, R. S., Fiser, R. H., Atkinson, R. L. & Carrel, R. E. The Prader–Willi syndrome: a study of 40 patients and a review of the literature. *Medicine* **62** (1983), 59–80.

15. Bartolucci, G. & Younger, J. Tentative classification of neuropsychiatric disturbances in Prader–Willi syndrome. *Journal of Intellectual Disability Research* **38** (1994), 621–629.

16. Clarke, D. J. Prader–Willi syndrome and psychotic symptoms: 2. A preliminary study of prevalence using the Psychopathology Assessment Schedule for Adults with Developmental Disability checklist. *Journal of Intellectual Disability Research* **42** (1998), 451–454.

17. Clarke, D., Boer, H., Webb, T. *et al*. Prader–Willi syndrome and psychotic symptoms 1. Case descriptions and genetic studies. *Journal of Intellectual Disability Research* **42** (1998), 440–450.

18. Verhoeven, W. M. A., Curfs, L. M. G. O. & Tuinier, S. Prader–Willi syndrome and cycloid psychoses. *Journal of Intellectual Disability Research* **42** (1998), 455–462.

19. World Health Organization. *The ICD-10 Classification of Mental and Behavioural Disorders*. Geneva: WHO, 1992.

20. Vogels, A., Matthijs, G., Legius, E., Devriendt, K. & Fryns, J. P. Chromosome 15 maternal uniparental disomy and psychosis in Prader–Willi syndrome. *Journal of Medical Genetics* **40** (2003), 72–73.

21. Gratacos, M., Nadal, M., Martin-Santos, R. *et al*. A polymorphic genomic duplication on human chromosome 15 is a susceptibility factor for panic and phobic disorders. *Cell* **106** (2001), 367–379.

22. Collier, D. A. FISH, flexible joints and panic: are anxiety disorders really expressions of instability in the human genome? *British Journal of Psychiatry* **181** (2002), 457–459.

23. Ewald, H., Mors, O., Flint, T. & Kruse, T. A. Linkage analysis between manic-depressive illness and the region on chromosome 15q involved in Prader–Willi syndrome, including two GABA(A) receptor subtype genes. *Human Heredity* **44** (1994), 287–294.

24. Papadimitriou, G. N., Dikeos, D. G., Karadima, G. *et al.* Association between the GABA(A) receptor alpha5 subunit gene locus (GABRA5) and bipolar affective disorder. *American Journal of Medical Genetics* **81** (1998), 73–80.

25. Turecki, G., Grof, P., Grof, E. *et al.* Mapping susceptibility genes for bipolar disorder: a pharmacogenetic approach based on excellent response to lithium. *Molecular Psychiatry* **6** (2001), 570–578.

26. Riley, B. P., Makoff, A., Mogudi-Carter, M. *et al.* Haplotype transmission disequilibrium and evidence for linkage of the CHRNA7 gene region to schizophrenia in Southern African Bantu families. *American Journal of Medical Genetics* **96** (2000), 196–201.

27. Freedman, R., Leonard, S., Olincy, A. *et al.* Evidence for the multigenic inheritance of schizophrenia. *American Journal of Medical Genetics* **105** (2001), 794–800.

28. Liu, C. M., Hwu, H. G., Lin, M. W. *et al.* Suggestive evidence for linkage of schizophrenia to markers at chromosome 15q13–14 in Taiwanese families. *American Journal of Medical Genetics* **105** (2001), 658–661.

29. Meyer, J., Ortega, G., Schraut, K. *et al.* Exclusion of the neuronal nicotinic acetylcholine receptor alpha7 subunit gene as a candidate for catatonic schizophrenia in a large family supporting the chromosome 15q13–22 locus. *Molecular Psychiatry* **7** (2002), 220–223.

30. Taylor, M., Bhagwagar, Z., Cowen, P. J. & Sharp, T. GABA and mood disorders. *Psychological Medicine* **33** (2003), 387–393.

31. Calzolari, E., Aiello, V., Palazzi, P. *et al.* Psychiatric disorder in a familial 15;18 translocation and sublocalization of myelin basic protein of 18q22.3. *American Journal of Medical Genetics* **67** (1996), 154–161.

32. Gillberg, C., Steffenburg, S., Wahlstrom, J. *et al.* Autism associated with marker chromosome. *Journal of the American Academy of Child and Adolescent Psychiatry* **30** (1991), 489–494.

33. Craddock, N. & Lendon, C. Chromosome Workshop: 11, 14 and 15. *American Journal of Medical Genetics (Neuropsychiatric Genetics)* **88** (1999), 244–254.

34. Silverstone, T., McPherson, H., Li, Q. & Doyle, T. Deep white matter hyperintensities in patients with bipolar depression, unipolar depression and age-matched control subjects. *Bipolar Disorders* **5** (2003), 53–57.

35. Moore, P. B., Shepherd, D. J., Eccleston, D. *et al.* Cerebral white matter lesions in bipolar affective disorder: relationship to outcome. *British Journal of Psychiatry* **178** (2001), 172–176.

36. Whittington, J. E., Holland, A. J., Webb, T., Butler, J. V., Clarke, D. J. & Boer, H. Cognitive abilities and genotype in a population-based sample of people with Prader–Willi syndrome. *Journal of Intellectual Disability Research* **48** (2003), 172–187.

37. Takhar, J. & Malla, A. K. Traitement a la Clozapine d'une psychose et du Parkinsonisme dans un cas phenotypique de syndrome de Praser–Willi. *Canadian Journal of Clinical Pharmacology* **4** (1997), 79–81.

11

Obsessions and compulsions

Several psychiatric conditions have been associated with PWS. As noted in Chapter 10, increased risk rates have been proposed for psychotic illness and obsessive–compulsive disorder (OCD). This chapter is concerned with the latter. Obsessive–compulsive behaviour has long been recognised as part of the PWS phenotype and it is generally agreed that people with PWS have 'obsessive personalities', but this is not the same as OCD.

While some reports on the obsessive–compulsive behaviour in PWS have raised the possibility of heightened rates of OCD in this population,[1,2,3] the difficulties of psychiatric diagnosis in people with learning disabilities (LD) seem to have discouraged attempts at quantification in PWS, although there are several estimates of prevalence in undifferentiated groups of people with LD.[4,5,6,7] Exceptionally, the 1996 paper by Dykens, Leckman & Cassidy[3] does seek to elucidate the nature of the obsessive–compulsive behaviour by people with PWS. We describe this paper in detail since, as well as being the most thorough investigation of obsessive–compulsive behaviour in PWS of the last decade, it raises several interesting issues.

In DSM-IV[8] a diagnosis of OCD presumes the presence of either obsessions (intrusive, recurrent thoughts or images that exceed real-life worries) or compulsions (repetitive behaviours that a person is driven to perform in response to an obsessional thought or set of rigid rules). Such behaviours serve to prevent or reduce distress and are time-consuming or significantly interfere with normal social, academic or occupational functioning. The onset is usually relatively sudden and the person has insight into their condition. Dykens, Leckman & Cassidy[3] report on 91 people with PWS, age range 5–47 years (mean 19), IQ range 50–89 (mean 69), recruited at a PWSA meeting, through PWSA family support groups, and through a PWSA publication. They also recruited 43 people without LD but with clinical OCD, from three clinics for OCD, matched to 43 of the PWS group by age and gender. For the PWS group, they used an informant version of the Yale–Brown Obsessive–Compulsive Scale[9] (Y-BOCS), which was completed at leisure by the main caregiver. For the OCD group, they used a self-report version. In both versions, 56 symptoms were either rated as being present in the last week, or ever (the former rating was used in the analyses). Ten additional Y-BOCS items were used to assess symptom severity, including the extent to which obsessions and compulsions were time-consuming, distressful, out of one's control and/or cause social or occupational impairment. Because a core symptom of PWS is obsessive–compulsive eating behaviour, the Y-BOCS items were restricted to non-food issues. The Y-BOCS scoring incorporates the diagnostic criteria for OCD that allows the extraction of a 'likely OCD' diagnosis. This was used in this paper.

Informants reported compulsions of 'hoarding and 'needing to tell or ask' (e.g. repetitive questioning) in over half of those with PWS (58%, 53%); ordering or arranging and repeating rituals were reported for 37–38%; cleaning (24%), counting (17%) and checking (15%) were other reported compulsions. Reporting of obsessions followed a similar pattern, but with lower rates. Informants estimated that compulsive behaviours resulted in 'moderate' to 'severe' distress in 64% of people with PWS, adaptive impairment in 80% and excessive time-consumption in 45%, as rated according to the Y-BOCS scales. A rating of 'moderate' is given if: 'reports that anxiety would mount but remain manageable if compulsions were prevented, or that anxiety increases but remains manageable during the performance of compulsions' (distress); 'there is definite interference with social or occupational performance, but still manageable' (adaptive impairment); 'spends from 1–3 hrs/day performing compulsions or frequent performance of compulsive behaviours (time-consuming)'.

Comparisons between PWS and OCD groups indicated significant ($P < 0.01$) differences for three compulsive behaviours; the PWS group showed more hoarding (79% v. 7%) and needing to tell or ask (51% v. 23%), but less checking behaviour (16% v. 55%). Other rates of compulsive behaviours did not differ significantly ($P > 0.05$). The authors concluded that the 'increased risks of OCD are strongly indicated in people with PWS, based on the range and severity of symptoms encountered in this sample'. This conclusion was moderated by their observation that formal diagnoses of OCD cannot be made on the basis of informant checklist ratings. However, they also pointed out that in the study, the pattern of symptoms in people with PWS indicated that these symptoms loaded on only one dimension of OCD, that is the principle factor extracted from a factor analysis of the Y-BOCS using data from 107 OCD patients.[10] Introducing the issue of cognitive limitations, they further noted that compulsive symptoms in those with PWS are remarkably similar to rituals and repetitive behaviours that are highly prevalent among normally developing preschool children.[11] The obsessive-compulsive behaviour in PWS, therefore, may be viewed as consistent with their 'mental age'. They used this argument to explain why people with PWS so affected do not appear to have insight into their symptoms and pointed out that DSM-IV allows this criterion to be dropped in the case of children. The factor loading of symptoms on a single dimension in a sample of people with PWS was confirmed in a 1998 report[12] of a factor analysis of Compulsive Behaviour Checklist scores. This factor analysis yielded only one general factor, with the exception of an item relating to 'deviant skin-grooming – skin-picking'.

We next consider findings on obsessions and compulsions from the Cambridge study of PWS. Most of the people in this study had never needed to seek help for any of the psychiatric conditions mentioned in the introduction, and none had sought help for, or been diagnosed as having, OCD. For this part of the study 87 people with PWS aged 5 years and over were included. Although the main instrument for assessing OCD in previous reports has been the Y-BOCS, we decided that it was inappropriate for our population study. First, like the ICD-10[13] and DSM-IV criteria, it requires that the person has insight enough to be distressed by his or her obsessions and/or compulsions. This is unlikely in people with LD and younger children. Our population sample of people with PWS covered all age groups and some had severe LD. Our assessment of the presence and extent of obsessions and compulsions in this population, therefore, had to be based on behavioural measures. Second, most psychiatric diagnoses require a clear onset and/or discrete episodes, whereas, in PWS, parental reports often indicate that the behaviour has been manifest 'always'. This seems to imply a pervasive personality trait, so we felt that it might be more appropriate to consider the behaviour as relating to obsessive–compulsive personality, rather than OCD. Rather than having a checklist, we asked general questions about behaviour in a semi-structured interview (usually 2.5 to 4 hours) with the main carer; in particular, we encouraged informants to describe all behaviours that they saw as problems. The main questionnaire covered the Consensus Diagnostic Criteria, behavioural symptoms, eating behaviour (including hoarding of objects as well as food), and childhood traits (attention deficit disorder, hyperactivity, autistic traits). We also administered the informant versions of the Development Behaviour Checklist (DBC) or the Aberrant Behaviour Checklist (ABC), depending on age, and the Vineland Adaptive Behaviour Scales. Anecdotes and explanations were encouraged throughout the interview, and follow-up questions were frequently used to elucidate ambiguous statements. One of the researchers also spent time (usually 90 minutes or more) with the person with PWS, administering the appropriate Wechsler ability scales and tests of attainment. This gave her opportunity to observe how the person coped with the situation, how they interacted with an authority figure in a one-to-one situation, and how well they attended to the tasks. The same two people conducted all of these interviews and tests.

Because of the eating disturbance in PWS, food obsessions were excluded from our enquiry: almost all of the people with PWS who were included in our study

Table 11.1. Characteristics of Prader–Willi syndrome (PWS) and comparison learning disabilities (LD) groups

	PWS group	LD group
Age (years) band		
0–15	33	22
16–30	40	9
31 +	24	12
Mean age (SD)	20.8 (12.5)	20.2 (14.6)
IQ band		
0–50	16	9
51–60	20	9
61–70	26	8
71–80	17	5
80 +	6	9
Mean IQ	63 (12.3)	64 (17.7)
Mean BMI	31.6 (11.8)	28.3 (10.1)

BMI: Body Mass Index.

appeared to spend a great deal of time thinking about food. Some had channelled their interest into courses on catering and cooking, some spent a lot of their time looking at cookery books, others just watched for opportunities to get their hands on food, or clock-watched from one meal to the next. This excessive interest in food was by far the most common obsessive–compulsive behaviour observed during our visits.

The comparison group with LD consisted of a combination of the PWS-like group and the recruited people with LD. The learning disabled, PWS-like, and PWS groups had similar mean age, mean IQ and mean BMI, as shown in Table 11.1. As noted in previous chapters, the same instruments and procedures were used for both groups. This means that we were able to estimate the prevalence of obsessive and compulsive symptoms associated with PWS, rather than with obesity or intellectual disability.

Two measures of compulsive symptoms were formed: *a simple count of the number of symptoms* from the list in Table 11.2, plus 'Needs routine' and 'Anticipation' that were endorsed by informants, and *a weighted count*, in which those behaviours rated as a severe problem were counted double. *Severity of eating behaviour* was rated separately. The sample was divided into the *age groups* 5–12, 13–19, 20+ years, corresponding roughly to childhood, adolescence, and adulthood. *IQ* was the full-scale score on the age-appropriate Wechsler ability tests. *Socialisation age*

Table 11.2. Obsessive–compulsive symptoms rated very frequent or very severe

	PWS[a] ($n = 93$)		PWSpop[b] ($n = 68$)		LD ($n = 42$)		χ^2 1 d.f.	P
	n^c	(%)	n^c	(%)	n^c	(%)		
Need to ask or tell	36/78	(46.2)	27/55	(49.1)	4/29	(13.8)	9.4	<0.01
Routines	26/80	(32.5)	17/57	(29.8)	4/33	(12.1)	5.0	<0.05
Hoarding	19/80	(23.7)	12/57	(21.1)	1/33	(3.0)	6.9	<0.01
Repetitive	18/80	(22.5)	14/57	(24.6)	3/33	(9.1)	2.8	NS
Ordering	11/80	(13.7)	11/57	(19.3)	0		5.0	<0.05
Cleaning	2/80	(2.3)	1/57	(1.8)	0		0.9	NS
Counting	0		0		0			NS
Checking	0		0		0			NS

[a] Total Prader–Willi syndrome (PWS) group.
[b] People with PWS in the population sample.
[c] The value of n varies because not all items are appropriate to all participants (e.g. those without speech).

was the age-equivalent score on the Socialisation subscale of the Vineland Adaptive Behaviour Scales. *Mood swings* were assessed by a composite of the sum of scores on our own questionnaire 'Mood swings – ever' (carer rating 0–4), and the score on the ABC (adults) or DBC (children) for the item 'Mood changes rapidly for no apparent reason'. *Anxiety or depression* was assessed by the sum of five scores on our PWS questionnaire, the items 'Ever had severe anxiety lasting more than a few days', 'Ever had severe depression lasting more than a few days', 'Ever had other nervous problem lasting more than a few days'; and on the Vineland Mal-adaptive Behaviour scale, the item 'Exhibits excessive unhappiness'; and on the ABC (adults) or DBC (children) on the item 'Depressed mood'. *Autistic traits* were assessed by the sum of scores on our screen of eight items (hardly ever: initiates con-versation, calls attention to things, smiles in response, co-operates in play, makes eye contact, shows imaginative play; but has repetitive talk, has little emotional expression).

Three interpretations of the obsessive–compulsive behaviour observed in PWS were considered in our analyses: the behaviour is compatible with high rates of OCD in the PWS population; the behaviour is compatible with a developmental delay; and the behaviour is compatible with arrested development. The first interpretation would imply that many people with PWS meet clinical criteria for OCD and, in particular, we might have expected symptoms to increase with age corresponding to onset times; the second interpretation would imply that the behaviour is related to (declines with) age and, possibly, IQ, if delay is dependent on mental age; while the third would imply that the behaviour is typical of that of a normal stage of development, perhaps dependent on IQ, and remains at a similar level, independent of age. Prior to analyses relevant to these interpretations, we contrasted the prevalence and severity of symptoms in the PWS and LD groups.

The prevalence rates of various symptoms are shown in Table 11.2. These rates were similar in the combined groups of people with PWS and in the population-based group. Prevalence in the PWS group significantly exceeded that in the LD group for the symptoms: *need to ask or tell, routines, hoarding* and *ordering*. No counting or checking symptoms were rated very frequent or severe in either group.

Compulsive symptoms did not increase or decline with *age* in the group with PWS and were not correlated with obesity (*BMI*), with (long-term) *anxiety/depression*, or with *severity of eating behaviour*. There were significant positive correlations with (short-term) *mood swings* ($R = 0.23$, $P = 0.05$ for *weighted compulsion count*) and *autistic symptoms* ($R = 0.52$, $P = 0.001$ for *weighted compulsion count*). There were significant negative correlations with *IQ* ($R = -0.30$, $P = 0.008$ for *weighted count*) and *socialisation age* ($R = -0.30$, $P = 0.002$ for *weighted count*). The correlation with *mood swings* was no longer significant when correction was applied for the number of contrasts. When the remaining significant correlations were re-examined in turn, controlling for the others, the only significant one was between *weighted compulsion count* and *autistic symptoms* ($R = 0.34$, $P = 0.005$), controlling for *IQ* and *socialisation age*. No significant correlations were found for the LD group.

A few stereotyped and ritualistic behaviours were seen during direct observation of the PWS participants. No tics were noted. Compulsive symptoms, however, were found to be much more prevalent in our PWS groups than in the comparison group of people with similar intellectual disabilities, who were of similar ages and had high BMIs. It is therefore unlikely that the high rate of compulsive symptoms in PWS is accounted for by their relative obesity or their intellectual disability.

The results of the Cambridge study of compulsive symptoms associated with PWS are broadly in agreement with the earlier study by Dykens *et al.*[3] Very few obsessional thoughts were reported and the range of compulsive symptoms described was relatively restricted, with few symptoms of counting, cleaning or checking. The prevalence of obsessional disorders, as distinct from compulsive acts, has been estimated at between 0.2% and 12% of clinical populations of children and adolescents.[14, 15] The pattern of compulsive symptoms observed in our data is similar to that seen in early childhood. Indeed, a combination of PWS behaviours, including labile mood, temper tantrums, ritualistic and compulsive symptoms, repetitive questions and insistence on routine are very similar to those of normally developing children in early childhood. In PWS, many of these behaviours persist into adulthood and throughout life. The prevalence of obsessional and compulsive symptoms varies throughout normal childhood. Bedtime and dressing rituals are common in early childhood.[16] After the emergence of repetitive behaviours, 'just right' behaviours are seen, such as having unique places for objects or lining things up in a certain way.[11] This, in turn, is followed by a phase of collecting or hoarding objects. When we looked at prevalence of individual symptoms with age in the PWS group, the only clear change was the decline of 'need to ask or tell' and the increase in 'hoarding' with increasing age. In a study of normal children aged one to six years,[11] compulsive behaviour, measured by the Child Routines Inventory, had higher rates in two- to four-year-olds than in younger or older children. Using the Maudsley Obsessive–Compulsive Inventory for a study of 1083 schoolchildren aged 8–13 years in Jerusalem,[17] it was found that obsessional ideas and compulsive behaviours were common among the younger children (eight years) but were present in only a minority at the age of 13 years. In our study, the lack of change in symptoms with age clearly neither supports the OCD nor the delayed development hypotheses, but rather is consistent with a specific pattern of arrested development. This latter hypothesis is also consistent with our observations of negative correlations with IQ and socialisation age, since in normally developing children the obsessive–compulsive phase declines from a peak between the ages of two and four years. The average age equivalent of our population PWS sample on the Vineland Interpersonal Relations Subscale was about 4.7 years, ranging from under two years to 14 years, while standard scores on the socialisation domain ranged from below 20 to 75 years.

We have already noted some of the arguments against an interpretation of the obsessive–compulsive behaviour in PWS as indicating high rates of OCD. In particular, the lack of a sudden onset and the loading on a single factor. A further argument comes from a comparison of our findings with a study of the presenting symptoms among 70 consecutive children and adolescents with a primary diagnosis of OCD.[18] This study found the most common obsessions to be those concerning contamination by dirt or germs (40%), worries about something terrible happening (24%), and worries about symmetry, order and exactness (17%). The most commonly reported compulsions were those concerning excessive or ritualised hand-washing, showering, bathing, tooth-brushing or grooming (85%), and repeating rituals such as going in and out of a doorway (51%) and checking compulsions (46%). Compulsions regarding ordering or arranging were found in 17%, counting in 18% and hoarding or collecting in 6%. These are similar in nature to those found in adult OCD and quite dissimilar to those in our PWS group.

The rates of compulsive symptoms are very high in our PWS groups, higher than in our contrast group of people with LD. People with PWS are also likely to become distressed, succumbing to temper tantrums, if their compulsive behaviours are prevented, for example by a break in routine. Do people with PWS, then, show any similarities with people diagnosed as having OCD that may suggest any common aetiology? The response of OCD to antidepressants such as clomipramine and specific serotonin reuptake inhibitors, as well as evidence from neurochemical studies, suggests the involvement of the serotonergic system in the genesis or maintenance of OCD.[18,19,20,21] Although abnormalities in serotonergic systems seem to play a part in the genesis of some OCDs, it seems likely that the anti-obsessional effect of drugs acting on serotonergic systems may result from alterations in the balance between serotonin and other neurotransmitters, or changes in receptor functioning.[22] One study has reported abnormal serotonin turnover associated with PWS, with increased concentrations of serotonin metabolites in the cerebrospinal fluid of children and adolescents with PWS compared with contrast groups.[23] Leckman *et al.*[23] reported elevated cerebrospinal fluid oxytocin concentrations is associated with OCD in people without intellectual disability. A reduction in the number of oxytocin-containing neurones in the paraventricular nucleus of the hypothalamus has been found in post-mortem studies of some people with PWS.[25]

There were no differences in mean number of compulsive symptoms in our full PWS sample between the two genetic subtypes, whether we looked at a simple count of symptoms or at a weighted count. We conclude that OCD in people with PWS is best conceptualised as arrested development. The implications of such a conclusion is that antidepressant medication (as used in true OCD) is less likely to be helpful for the treatment of these obsessions and rituals and that management requires behavioural strategies that minimise the risk of positive reinforcement of such behaviours and that helps occupy the person with PWS so that routines and rituals do not become established in a manner that impinges on his or her quality of life.

REFERENCES

1. Hellings, J. A. & Warnock, J. K. Self-injurious behaviour and serotonin in Prader–Willi syndrome. *Psychopharmacology Bulletin* **30** (1994), 245–250.
2. Stein, D. J., Hollander, E., Simeon, D. & Cohen, L. Impulsivity scores in patients with obsessive–compulsive disorder. *Journal of Nervous and Mental Disease* **182** (1994), 240–241.
3. Dykens, E. M., Leckman, J. F. & Cassidy, S. B. Obsessions and compulsions in Prader–Willi syndrome. *Journal of Child Psychology and Psychiatry* **37** (1996), 995–1002.
4. Meyers, B. A. Psychopathology in hospitalized developmentally disabled individuals. *Comprehensive Psychiatry* **27** (1986), 115–126.
5. Meyers, B. A. Psychiatric problems in adolescents with developmental disabilities. *Journal of the American Academy of Child and Adolescent Psychiatry* **26** (1987), 74–79.

6. Menolascino, F. L., Levitas, A. & Greiner, C. The nature and types of mental illness in the mentally retarded. *Psychopharmacology Bulletin* **22** (1986), 1060–1071.

7. Vitiello, B., Spreat, S. & Behar, D. Obsessive Compulsive Disorder in mentally retarded patients. *Journal of Nervous and Mental Disease* **177** (1989), 232–236.

8. American Psychiatric Association. *Diagnostic and Statistical Manual of Mental Disorders*, 4th edn. Washington, DC: American Psychiatric Association, 1994.

9. Goodman, W. K., Price, L. H., Rasmussen, S. A. *et al.* The Yale–Brown Obsessive Compulsive Scale. Part 1: Development, use and reliability. *Archives of General Psychiatry* **46** (1989), 1006–1011.

10. Baer, L. Factor analysis of symptom subtypes of obsessive–compulsive disorder and their relation to personality and tic disorders. *Journal of Clinical Psychiatry* **55** (1993), 18–23.

11. Evans, D. W., Leckman, J. F. & Carter, A. Ritual, habit and perfectionism: the prevalence and development of compulsive-like behaviour in normal young children. *Child Development* **68** (1997), 56–68.

12. Feurer, L. D., Dimitropoulos, A., Stone, W. L. *et al.* The latent variable structure of the Compulsive Behaviour Checklist in people with Prader–Willi syndrome. *Journal of Intellectual Disability Research* **42** (1998), 472–480.

13. World Health Organization. *The ICD-10 Classification of Mental and Behavioural Disorders*. Geneva: WHO, 1992.

14. Judd, L. Obsessive–Compulsive neurosis in children. *Archives of General Psychiatry* **12** (1965), 136–143.

15. Hollingsworth, C. E., Tanguay, P. E., Grossman, L. *et al.* Long-term outcome of obsessive–compulsive disorders in childhood. *Journal of the American Academy of Child and Adolescent Psychiatry* **19** (1980), 134–144.

16. Gesell, A., Ames, L. B. & Ilg, F. L. *The Infant and the Child in Culture Today*. New York: Harper & Row, 1974.

17. Zohar, A. H. & Bruno, R. Normative and pathological obsessive–compulsive behaviour and ideation in childhood: a question of timing. *Journal of Child Psychology and Psychiatry* **38** (1997), 993–999.

18. Goodman, W. K. *et al.* Pharmacologic challenges in obsessive–compulsive disorder. In Zohar, J., Insel, T. & Rasmussen, S. (Eds). *The Psychology of Obsessive–Compulsive Disorder*, pp. 162–186. New York: Springer, 1991.

19. Riddle, M. A., Scahill, L., King, R. A. *et al.* Double-blind crossover trial of fluoxetine and placebo in children and adolescents with obsessive–compulsive disorder. *Journal of the American Academy of Child and Adolescent Psychiatry* **31** (1992), 1062–1069.

20. Zohar, J., Mueller, E. A., Insel, T. R. *et al.* Serotonergic responsivity in obsessive–compulsive disorder: comparison of patients and health controls. *Archives of General Psychiatry* **44** (1987), 946–951.

21. Zohar, J., Insel, T., Zohar-Kadouch, R. *et al.* Serotonergic responsivity in obsessive–compulsive disorder: effects of chronic clomipramine treatment. *Archives of General Psychiatry* **45** (1988), 167–172.

22. Murphy, D., Zohar, J., Pato, M. *et al.* Obsessive–compulsive disorder as a 5-HT subsystem-related behavioural disorder. *British Journal of Psychiatry* **155** (Suppl. 8) (1989), 15–24.

23. Akefeldt, A., Ekman, R., Gillberg, C. *et al.* Cerebrospinal fluid monoamines in Prader–Willi syndrome. *Biological Psychiatry* **44** (1998), 1321–1328.

24. Leckman, J. F., Goodman, W. K., North, W. G. *et al.* Elevated cerebrospinal fluid level of oxytocin in obsessive-compulsive disorder. *Archives of General Psychiatry* **51** (1994), 782–792.

25. Swaab, D. F., Purba, J. S. & Hofman, M. A. Alterations in the hypothalamic paraventricular nucleus and its oxytocin neurons (putative satiety cells) in Prader–Willi syndrome: a study of five cases. *Journal of Clinical Endocrinology and Metabolism* **80** (1995), 573–579.

Part III

Minor findings, some conclusions and future directions

12

Understanding PWS

In the previous chapters we examined different aspects of PWS drawing upon anecdotal information, previously published research and systematically collected data from our Cambridge population-based study, to help clarify and illuminate particular issues. Whilst a considerable amount is now known about the syndrome, some of the most crucial aspects still remain elusive. Most striking is whether it is caused by the absence of expression of one or more genes, and which genes. What is clear is that these genes are normally only expressed when inherited from the father, being imprinted when inherited from the mother. At present the SnoRNAs are the main candidates, but until this is fully elucidated, it is not possible to say what the 'PWS gene(s)' do and therefore what does not happen when they are not expressed. The second area that remains a considerable mystery is the mechanisms that provide the link between the abnormal gene expression (genotype) and the physical and behavioural phenotype. The crucial issue here is whether all that is characteristic of people with PWS can be explained by one mechanism (and by implication the absence of expression of one gene) or whether more than one underlying process is necessary to explain the full phenotype (and by implication absence of expression of more than one gene).

In this final chapter, first, we consider some of the other issues in the literature that could possibly have a bearing on PWS. Second, we reconsider aspects of our own and other research, for which we have no explanation at present, and which may or may not eventually prove to be relevant to the future understanding of PWS. The chapter ends by considering future directions in PWS research.

Other findings

Set out below, we briefly cover other observations not considered elsewhere that either require explanation or have implications for support services.

Autism and PWS

There is a body of literature linking autism with abnormalities (mainly multiple copies of sections of genetic material) of chromosome 15[1,2,3,4] and it has been proposed that this might give rise to differences in the prevalence rates of autism in the main genetic subtypes of PWS.[4,5] Our screen for autistic traits, admittedly a basic screen, did not show any differences between the subtypes. In a study designed to detect such differences, there was no significant difference between the genetic subtypes in rates above the threshold on the Autism Screening Questionnaire, although the disomy group had higher total scores.[5] It seems likely that multiple extra copies of parts of the maternal chromosome 15 are implicated in autism, but people with PWS are not otherwise at risk.

Dyslexia and PWS

Dyslexia has also occasionally been linked to chromosome 15,[6] and at least one study of people with PWS has reported high levels of dyslexia.[7] However, linkage studies have pointed to a region of chromosome 15 outside the PWS region, q21–q22, as being most promising.[8,9] Moreover, as our research described in Chapter 7 shows, people with PWS of both main genetic types have higher attainment in reading than in other areas. On average, the people with the disomy form of PWS in our sample were reading at a level appropriate to their general ability (IQ). Again, we suggest that people with PWS are no more at risk of dyslexia than the general population.

Panic and anxiety disorders and PWS

Panic disorder has been linked to a locus on chromosome 15. Through the co-occurrence of panic and phobic disorders with joint laxity an interstitial duplication of chromosome 15q24–q26 (named *DUP25*) has been found to be significantly associated with panic/agoraphobia/social phobia/joint laxity in families and with panic disorder in non-familial cases.[10] Mosaicism in some affected people and different forms of *DUP25* within the same family, together with a finding of *DUP25* in 7% of a comparison group, indicates that *DUP25* is a susceptibility factor for a clinical phenotype that includes panic and phobic disorders, and joint laxity. Possibly the development of the disorder is gene dose dependent. So far no candidate gene has been identified among the 60 or so genes in the duplicated region.[11] In general, people with PWS have low levels of anxiety and are not at risk for panic or phobic disorder.

Severe weight loss in PWS

Turning to observations arising from the Cambridge project, perhaps the most intriguing concerns a number of people with PWS who, having successfully completed a carefully monitored programme of weight loss, have failed to stop losing weight when given an increased diet to maintain a target weight. We have now heard of six such people, all men, at least one of whom was hospitalised as a result of the continuing weight loss. We cannot explain why this should occur at all, or why all have been male.

Clinical/genetic discrepancies

Another observation that needs to be explained concerns the occasional person in whom clinical and genetic findings are at odds, in particular, case studies 1 and 2 from Chapter 5. Both of these people show normal methylation at the informative *SNRPN* locus; one has a deletion at 15q12, the other no obvious abnormality, but both have high scores on the clinical diagnostic criteria. There are two potential explanations. First, a single gene mutation of the 'PWS gene', ruled out by most of the experts in the genetics of PWS, could explain such examples (see below). Second, there may be another disorder, probably genetically determined, that has a very similar phenotype to PWS, but a genotype that has a different chromosomal locus. Once the probable 'PWS gene' is identified, sequencing studies of the genes from the DNA of these clinically positive but genetically negative cases, looking for mutations, would be indicated.

Parenting and carer stress

Much of the focus of research and of this book has been to explain how the PWS genotype might result in a particular pattern of development and cluster of problems. However, in the field of learning disabilities, applied behavioural analysis has shown how behaviours can be shaped by the responses of others. Although the propensity to a particular type of behaviour may be largely biologically determined, its frequency and severity may clearly depend on how others support a person with PWS and respond to such behaviours when they occur. From a different perspective, many of the anecdotes told to us during the course of the research indicated just how problematic it could be trying to cope with some aspects of the behaviour of a person with PWS, such as repetitive questioning or temper outbursts.

We have been able to find only one investigation into parenting styles in PWS.[12] This investigation showed that, compared with parents of people with Fragile X or Williams syndrome, parents of people with PWS have higher levels of stress that result in more anger towards their child, more parental inconsistency and worse child behaviour. Our own informal observations were that, however achieved, rigid adherence to (formal or informal) rules correlated with better behaviour from the PWS child, while inconsistent adherence to rules correlated with worse behaviour. However, in a cross-sectional study it was impossible to determine which came first, or whether there was a causal connection.

We used the Rutter Malaise inventory[13] as a rough measure of carer stress. Such stress has been found to be greater in the carers of people with PWS than in carers of other learning disabled groups. Over 40% of parents and 40% of professional carers who completed the inventory had sought professional help for psychiatric symptoms. Of those who completed the inventory, 26.6% of parents and 35% of professional carers had 10 or more malaise symptoms. These figures compare with rates of depression of 3.7% among carers of people with learning disabilities in a survey in Leicestershire.[14] In two studies of stress in parents of children with PWS, high levels of stress were reported; one study compared parents of children with PWS with parents of children with a mixed aetiology of learning disabilities and found higher levels in the former,[15] the other study reported more than 70% of mothers of children with PWS as being in need of psychological counselling.[16]

Bruising in PWS

Anecdotally, several mothers of people with PWS reported that their sons or daughters bruised easily. We have not systematically recorded this information, but we have come to appreciate that it should be recorded and researched more thoroughly for the protection of parents, in view of the importance placed on signs of bruising in child abuse. Bruising may result from severe temper tantrums, in which the person with PWS may hit him or herself and head bang.

The future of PWS research

Although a rather simplistic perspective, it is perhaps helpful to consider three main areas of research. First, there is the genotype, second, there is the mediating mechanisms linking the genotype to the third area, that is the behavioural and physical phenotype. There is a danger that research remains within each of these boxes, rather than makes the necessary connections that will provide the important conceptual leap forward. Below, we review further research strategies, and end the chapter by putting forward a hypothetical model of PWS that attempts to unify the state of knowledge as it exists at present. The model may or may not be correct, but what it does is challenges some present conceptions and provides a framework for bringing together the three areas of work mentioned above.

Genetics and animal models of PWS

From the great strides, particularly in genetics, which have been made in PWS research in the past two decades, the future of one strand of PWS research is clear. More imprinted 'suspect PWS genes' will be identified in the PWS region and their gene products identified. For obvious reasons, it is difficult to determine the biological consequence that follows the absence of expression of such genes in humans, particularly when the organ concerned is the brain, but the creation of what are referred to as 'knockout' mouse models (mice bred with an induced abnormality of the putative PWS genes) will enable the testing of the relevant PWS genes. Through these types of approaches, the fundamentals of the syndrome will eventually be understood.

PWS was first described less than 50 years ago. The volume of research findings described in earlier chapters gives some idea of the knowledge accumulated about the syndrome in that relatively short time. Twenty years ago the disomy form of PWS had not been recognised, the PWS region had not been delineated, the relevance of imprinted genes and the imprinting centre, and mutations thereof, had not been discovered. Thus, the time-scale to a full understanding of the fundamental problem could be relatively short. More difficult to predict is the spin-off in terms of knowledge not directly related to that fundamental problem. We have already seen how the 'PWS diagnostic criterion' of *fair-for-family* is now interpreted as being a consequence, in the deletion and isodisomy forms of PWS only, of the loss of one allele of a pigmentation gene, thereby making inheritance of a recessive characteristic more probable. A similar phenomenon brought to light by the syndrome, but not intrinsic to it, is the finding described in Chapter 10 concerning disomy forms of PWS and psychosis. We speculate below on the nature of some of the possible spin-offs as well as describing the directions that the Cambridge group's continuing research is taking.

Clinical research

The main foci of our own research will be in four broad areas, three of which directly relate to the previous population-based study. The first is a further exploration of the relationship between PWS and psychotic illness. The second is to investigate the influence of cognitive function and some of the differences between genetic subtypes. The third is to follow up the original cohort to look at longitudinal changes in individuals. The fourth area is using Positron Emission Tomographic (PET) brain scanning to investigate the cerebral basis of satiety and how it might be faulty in PWS. These studies are summarised in Figure 12.1.

PWS and psychotic illness

The main aim of the psychosis study is to determine whether the age of onset and marked propensity to psychotic illness observed to affect those people with PWS resulting from maternal disomy of chromosome 15 is due to the effect of

Psychosis
- Verify findings regarding disomies
- If yes, characterise illness
- If no, estimate risk factors

Genetic investigation of
candidate imprinted genes

Genetics
Further investigation
of +ve clinical but -ve
genetic cases

Cognition
- Characterise deletion–disomy differences
- Estimate parent–child IQ correlations
- In disomies, mother–child ability matching

Cognitve study
using invoked potentials

Satiety
- Scanning study of hunger and satiation states
- PWS v. normal (v. anorexia?)
- How does pattern of brain activity change?

Ethical considerations

Investigation of first stage of PWS

Genetic investigation
of placental imprinted
genes

Characteristics of new-born PWS
- same/differ from stage 2?

Comparisons with
Small-for-dates babies

Wider collaborations

Collection of brain tissue   Mouse models   European research

Figure 12.1. Planned future studies of Prader–Willi syndrome (PWS).

one major gene, or is an interaction between different biological and/or socially determined factors leading to a shift in the liability threshold. In particular, we aim to characterise the phenomenology of the psychotic illness that has been observed in adults with PWS, to determine whether it differs depending on the genetic subtype of PWS (when it does occur in those with a deletion), and to refute or confirm our original prevalence findings: that *all* people with PWS due to maternal disomy of chromosome 15, or with an imprinting centre mutation, will develop a psychotic illness in early adult life (by about 30 years), but not those with PWS due to chromosome 15 deletion. Further, we aim to investigate other risk factors that influence age of onset and prevalence of psychiatric illness in PWS generally. We hypothesise that there will be different influences in the two genetic subtypes of PWS. The genetic model we have proposed to explain the 100% occurrence of psychotic illness affecting adults with PWS with disomy predicts that any familial genetic influence in this group as a whole would be predominately from either the maternal or paternal side, not from both. In contrast, we predict that familial loading for psychiatric disorder on either side of the family, and the level of disability, will be the best predictor of prevalence and age of onset of psychiatric disorder in those with deletion. We predict that those with disomy will be at particular risk of developing a psychotic illness in early adult life in the context of a major life event and/or dieting. There is evidence that, in the general population, dieting brings about change in mood.[17] People with PWS are often forced to diet in early adult life because of the life-threatening obesity that results at that time, with increasing independence and free access to food. We speculate that the occurrence of a major life event and/or dieting for those with disomy will precipitate the development of an affective psychotic illness and will be a significant determinant of age of onset of psychiatric disorder.

PWS and cognition

The cognitive research will first test the hypothesis that the normal distribution of scores on general intelligence found in our population-based sample of people with PWS is a function of the influence of parental IQ, as it is in the general population, with the shift downwards in mean IQ by 40 points being a direct effect of a maternally imprinted gene at the chromosomal locus 15q11–q13. Second, the research will investigate differences in the cognitive profiles of the two genetic subgroups, and will correlate such differences with specific parental cognitive abilities. We shall investigate whether the reported exceptional visuo-spatial skills in those with deletion, and the strong vocabulary skills reported to predominate in those with disomy, are functions of parental visuo-spatial and maternal language abilities, respectively. Ability differences between the genetic subtypes that cannot be explained by parental ability differences may be capable of a more global explanation, such as an imprinted gene that confers a preferential laterality difference in functioning, which might correlate with other laterality preferences, or with brain pathology, as was shown in a study of children with temporal lobe epilepsy.[18] The Cambridge team will therefore be looking at laterality preferences. Although not included in our proposed research, we note that the studies[19,20,21] of the PWS brain referenced in Chapter 2 could be extended to look at differences between the main genetic subtypes: are there differences in structural abnormalities,[19] NAA/(Cho+Cr) ratios,[20] or evoked potentials on different tasks[21]? Another more global explanation of PWS deletion–disomy differences in cognitive profile may lie in the suggestion of 'male' and 'female' brains,[22] the former typified as objective, rational and analytical, and the latter as emotional and nurturing. Thus the 'male' brain would excel at analytical puzzles, while the 'female' brain would excel at communication skills. Most people are hypothesised to have a mixture of these extremes, and maybe in PWS the genetic subtypes incline them towards different proportions. In this case we would expect that people with PWS due to chromosome 15 disomy would be better at judging emotions, and better at judging acceptable social behaviour. Few gender differences have been reported in PWS studies of cognition or behaviour; we propose to extend our own investigation of gender in PWS to play and leisure activities.

PWS and satiety

We propose to use PET activation studies to investigate the cerebral basis of the abnormal eating behaviour observed in people with PWS. The development of techniques for brain scanning reveals differential areas of activation when performing particular tasks,[23] suggesting that the satiety response might be localised in this way. This has now been shown in the first reported study[24] using normal participants. It was found that hunger, after a 36-hour fast, was associated with increased activity in the hypothalamus and insular cortex and in some paralimbic and limbic areas, whereas satiation, following a meal, was associated with increased activity in the ventromedial prefrontal cortex, dorsolateral prefrontal cortex and inferior parietal lobule. Further similar studies of people without PWS have confirmed differential activation patterns in the two states. We have hypothesised that in PWS activation patterns in the hunger state will be normal, but that normal activation patterns after an average meal will not be apparent, although we consider it is possible that the pattern may be invoked by an abnormally large food intake.

A hypothetical model to help conceptualise PWS?

As described at the beginning of this chapter, one of the most significant unanswered questions is how many maternal imprinted paternally expressed genes are involved? The many different characteristics of the phenotype might arise either as a result of a failure of expression, in those with the PWS genotype, of a combination of separate imprinted genes, or there may be a common mechanism that accounts for the phenotype and only one gene involved. The former type of hypothesis is against the scientific principle of parsimony and no single gene has yet been shown to affect just one, or even a small group of, PWS characteristics.

As explained in Chapter 8, our observations of people with PWS and information given to us by their main carers led us to propose that there is a core set of symptoms that are always present, another set for which, compared with the normal population, people with PWS experience a threshold shift that makes occurrence more likely, and a set of behaviours that appear to reflect arrested development, in that they are typical of a childhood stage of normal development. Thus, at most, three mechanisms are needed to explain the phenotype. Might it be possible, then, that each mechanism is under the control of a single gene, and that at most three genes are involved? Alternatively, can these all be regarded as aspects of a single mechanism? Is what we refer to as 'all-or-none' just a threshold shift to a point at the extreme of the normal distribution, and arrested development a threshold shift that places the threshold to further maturational development outside the PWS range?

Further reflection on the phenotype of PWS, together with the findings outlined in Chapter 2 of specific hormonal and other deficiencies concerned with energy balance, has led us to a more radical hypothesis that challenges two aspects of our current understanding. First, that paradoxically, this syndrome, often seen as a genetic model for obesity, should be re-conceptualised as a syndrome of starvation, that becomes manifest as obesity in a food rich environment. Second, although this syndrome is generally considered to be a contiguous gene disorder, the full phenotype may in fact be explained by the failure of expression of the paternal allele of a single maternally imprinted gene that has a controlling influence on energy balance. Some of the reasoning that led to this hypothesis is outlined below.

As noted in Chapter 1, PWS is characterised by two distinct phenotypes. During fetal life there is limited fetal movement, and at birth, evidence of fetal growth retardation and severe hypotonia. The infant fails to thrive and tube feeding is necessary. The second phenotype, described in most of the literature and in the foregoing chapters, begins at about two years of age, by which time weaning would normally have occurred. There is a marked propensity to excessive eating that continues throughout life, and obesity can only effectively be prevented by controlling access to food. The endophenotypic characteristics that require a unitary explanation if a single gene model is to be accepted are: the growth and gonadotrophin hormonal deficiencies (which account for the physical phenotype); the arrested brain development (which accounts for the learning disability and behaviour pattern); and the abnormal satiety response (which accounts for the obesity), together with the childhood characteristics of neonatal hypotonia and failure to thrive.

After food intake the levels of cholecystokinin, leptin, neuropeptide Y and agouti-related protein found in PWS (Chapter 2) would normally be associated with a state of satiation, but in PWS they clearly are not. Thus, the fundamental pathophysiological abnormality in PWS is that these particular peripheral and central influences do not lead to the metabolic and psychological changes (e.g. loss of hunger) controlled by the hypothalamus, that normally follow food intake. In PWS, because of the hypothesised interruption of the normal hypothalamic pathways (consequent upon the PWS genetic abnormality), the body incorrectly perceives itself to be in a state of starvation. As a result, the body's metabolic rate is reduced and gonadotrophin release is impaired, as in starvation states such as anorexia nervosa. Further support for the 'starvation' model comes from the observation that levels of the orexigenic hormone ghrelin are markedly elevated in people with PWS, compared to obese and non-obese non-PWS comparison groups,[25, 26] but they are also found to be elevated in people with anorexia nervosa.[27] Abnormally, ghrelin levels in PWS neither vary with food intake nor correlate with hunger ratings.[25] An observation that links eating and growth hormone (GH) secretion is that ghrelin is a ligand of the GH secretagogue receptor (GHS-R)[28] and stimulates GH releasing hormone (GHRH) and therefore GH release.[29] However, in PWS, contrary to expectation, high ghrelin levels are not associated with high or even normal levels of GH despite the presence of normal GHRH neurones.[30] This may be explained by the observation in rats that continuous stimulation by ghrelin results in the desensitisation of the GH secretory response.[31] We hypothesise that the desensitisation of GHS-R, due to chronically increased levels of ghrelin, is one possible explanation for the GH deficiency. The eating behaviour and the GH and gonadotrophin deficits (and thereby the physical phenotype) can therefore be explained by a single pathophysiological mechanism.

The aspects of the phenotype remaining to be explained are the neonatal hypotonia, failure to thrive and arrested brain development. Here we propose that the starvation model also applies to the early phenotype. We hypothesise that it is the absence of expression of the 'imprinted PWS gene' in the placenta that disrupts nutrition to the fetus, resulting in fetal starvation and abnormal brain development. A further factor may be the detrimental effects of low levels of GH and insulin-like growth hormone (IGF) on brain development[32] and on muscle mass in the fetus. During fetal life and up until weaning, growth is controlled by the mother through regulation across the placenta and, after birth, in terms of milk supply.[32] After weaning, control of energy balance is centrally regulated by the infant as described above. We know that PWS is caused by one or more imprinted genes and there is considerable evidence that imprinted genes are important in the control of fetal growth in placental mammals.[33]

We do not yet know which imprinted genes on chromosome 15 are expressed in the human placenta, nor have we been able to find studies of hormone concentrations (such as GH, ghrelin, or leptin) in PWS babies. However, all three have been studied in cord blood from normal babies at delivery.[34] The role of ghrelin in the placenta is not known, but leptin and leptin receptor integrity is considered important for placental function.[35] Indirect support for the deficit being placental, rather than fetal, in origin comes from the evidence of marked catch-up growth that occurs with augmented feeding immediately after birth.[36] The Cambridge team are setting up collaborative studies to address some of these issues.

Conclusion

The three main clinical advances that have had a significant impact on the lives of people with PWS and that of their families have, in our view, been the following. First, even though the actual gene or genes are not known, an early genetic diagnosis is now possible so that parents can be given an early explanation of their child's problems and can plan accordingly. Second, there is now a better understanding of the eating disorder in particular, and some of the other behavioural and physical phenotypic characteristics, so that appropriate strategies can be put into place to prevent obesity and to try and minimise and effectively manage some of the other problems. Third, the role of GH has been shown to go beyond simply improving height to influences on motivation, muscle strength and possibly general well-being. Another area of change that has been crucial has been the establishment of local, national and international support groups, and through them the dissemination of information. There is a sense that we are on the threshold of advances that will not only take us a conceptual leap forward but will also lead to new treatments. For example, if the fundamental abnormality that results in failure of satiety could be understood, pharmacological treatments might then become possible that would control the eating behaviour. Similarly, as the risk for psychotic illness becomes clearer, we will be in a better position to advise on its treatment. We therefore end this book on an optimistic note but in full appreciation of the difficulties that people with PWS and their families face.

REFERENCES

1. Demb, H. B. & Papola, P. PDD and Prader–Willi syndrome. *Journal of the American Academy of Child and Adolescent Psychiatry* **34** (1995), 539–540.
2. Descheemaeker, M. J., Vogels, A., Govers, V. *et al.* Prader–Willi syndrome: new insights in the behavioral and psychiatric spectrum. *Journal of Intellectual Disability Research* **46** (2002), 41–50.
3. Dykens, E. M. & Kasari, C. Maladaptive behavior in children with Prader–Willi syndrome, Down syndrome, and nonspecific mental retardation. *American Journal on Mental Retardation* **102** (1997), 228–237.
4. Veltman, M. W. M., Craig, E. E. & Bolton, P. F. Autism spectrum disorders in Prader–Willi and Angelman syndromes: a systematic review. (Unpublished data.)
5. Veltman, M. W. M., Thompson, R. J., Roberts, S. E. *et al.* Prader–Willi syndrome: a study comparing deletion and uniparental disomy cases. *European Child and Adolescent Psychiatry.* (In press.)
6. Boyar, F. Z., Whitney, M. M., Lossie, A. C. *et al.* A family with a grand-maternally derived interstitial duplication of proximal 15q. *Clinical Genetics* **60** (2001), 421–430.

7. Gross-Tsur, V., Landau, Y. E., Benarroch, F., Wertman-Elad, R. & Shalev, R. S. Cognition, attention, and behavior in Prader–Willi syndrome. *Journal of Child Neurology* **16** (2001), 288–290.

8. Nopola-Hemmi, J., Taipale, M., Haltia, T., Lehesjoki, A. E., Voutilainen, A. & Kere, J. Two translocations of chromosome 15q associated with dyslexia. *Journal of Medical Genetics* **37** (2000), 771–775.

9. Morris, D. W., Robinson, L., Turic, D. *et al.* Family-based association mapping provides evidence for a gene for reading disability on chromosome 15q. *Human Molecular Genetics* **9** (2000), 843–848.

10. Gratacos, M., Nadal, M., Martin-Santos, R. *et al.* A polymorphic genomic duplication on human chromosome 15 is a susceptibility factor for panic and phobic disorders. *Cell* **106** (2001), 367–379.

11. Collier, D. A. FISH, flexible joints and panic: are anxiety disorders really expressions of instability in the human genome? *British Journal of Psychiatry* **181** (2002), 457–459.

12. van Lieshout, C. F., De Meyer, R. E., Curfs, L. M. & Fryns, J. P. Family contexts, parental behaviour, and personality profiles of children and adolescents with Prader–Willi, Fragile-X, or Williams syndrome. *Journal of Child Psychology and Psychiatry* **39** (1998), 699–710.

13. Rutter, M. Malaise inventory. In Rutter, M., Tizard, J. & Whitmore, K. (Eds). *Education, health and behaviour*, Appendix 7. London: Longman, 1981.

14. McGrother, C. W., Hauck, A., Bhaumik, S., Thorp, C. & Taub, N. Community care for adults with learning disability and their carers: needs and outcomes from the Leicestershire register. *Journal of Intellectual Disability Research* **40** (1996), 183–190.

15. Hodapp, R. M., Dykens, E. M. & Masino, L. L. Families of children with Prader–Willi syndrome: stress-support and relations to child characteristics. *Journal of Autism and Developmental Disorders* **27** (1997), 11–24.

16. Sarimski, K. Psychological aspects of Prader–Willi syndrome. Results of a parent survey. [Article in German.] *Zeitschrift fur Kinder Jugendpsychiatri* **23** (1995), 267–274.

17. Anderson, I. M., Parry-Billings, M., Newsholme, E. A., Fairburn, C. G. & Cowen, P. J. Dieting reduces plasma tryptophan and alters brain 5-HT function in women. *Psychological Medicine* **20** (1990), 785–791.

18. Gadian, D. G., Isaacs, E. B., Cross, J. H. *et al.* Lateralization of brain function in childhood revealed by magnetic resonance spectroscopy. *Neurology* **46** (1996), 974–977.

19. Leonard, C. M., Williams, C. A., Nicholls, R. D. *et al.* Angelman and Prader–Willi syndrome: a magnetic resonance imaging study of differences in cerebral structure. *American Journal of Medical Genetics* **46** (1993), 26–33.

20. Hashimoto, T., Mori, K., Yoneda, Y. *et al.* Proton magnetic resonance spectroscopy of the brain in patients with Prader–Willi syndrome. *Pediatric Neurology* **18** (1998), 30–35.

21. Stauder, J. E., Brinkman, M. J. & Curfs, L. M. Multi-modal P3 deflation of event-related brain activity in Prader–Willi syndrome. *Neuroscience Letters* **327** (2002), 99–102.

22. Baron-Cohen, S. The extreme male brain theory of autism. *Trends in Cognitive Science* **6** (2002), 248–254.

23. Owen, A. M., Stern, C. E., Look, R. B., Tracey, I., Rosen, B. R. & Petrides, M. Functional organisation of spatial and non-spatial working memory processes within the human lateral frontal cortex. *Proceedings of the National Academy of Science of the USA* **95** (1998), 7721–7726.

24. Tataranni, P. A., Gautier, J.-F., Chen, K. *et al.* Neuroanatomical correlates of hunger and satiation in humans using positron emission tomography. *Proceedings of the National Academy of Science of the USA* **96** (1999), 4569–4574.

25. DelParigi, A., Tschop, M., Heiman, M. L. *et al.* High circulating ghrelin: a potential cause for hyperphagia and obesity in Prader–Willi syndrome. *Journal of Clinical Endocrinology and Metabolism* **87** (2002), 5461–5464.

26. Haqq, A. M., Farooqi, I. S., O'Rahilly, S. *et al.* Serum ghrelin levels are inversely correlated with body mass index, age, and insulin concentrations in normal children and are markedly increased in Prader–Willi syndrome. *Journal of Clinical Endocrinology and Metabolism* **88** (2003), 174–178.

27. Tolle, V., Kadem, M., Bluet-Pajot, M. T. *et al.* Balance in ghrelin and leptin plasma levels in anorexia nervosa patients and constitutionally thin women. *Journal of Clinical Endocrinology and Metabolism* **88** (2003), 109–116.

28. Kojima, M., Hosoda, H., Date, Y., Nakazato, M., Matsuo, H. & Kangawa, K. Ghrelin is a growth-hormone-releasing acylated peptide from stomach. *Nature* **402** (1999), 656–660.

29. Casanueva, F. F. & Dieguez, C. Ghrelin: the link connecting growth with metabolism and energy homeostasis. *Revues of Endocrine and Metabolic Disorders* **3** (2002), 325–338.

30. Goldstone, A. P., Unmehopa, U. A., Bloom, S. R. & Swaab, D. F. Hypothalamic NPY and agouti-related protein are increased in human illness but not in Prader–Willi syndrome and other obese subjects. *Journal of Clinical Endocrinology and Metabolism* **87** (2002), 927–937.

31. Date, Y., Murakami, N., Kojima, M. *et al.* Central effects of a novel acylated peptide, ghrelin, on growth hormone release in rats. *Biochemical and Biophysical Research Communications* **275** (2000), 477–480.

32. Lobie, P. E., Zhu, T., Graichen, R. & Goh, E. L. K. Growth hormone, insulin-like growth factor l and the CNS: localization, function and mechanism of action. *Growth Hormone and IGF Research* Suppl. B (2000), S51–S56.

33. Reik, W., Davies, K., Dean, W., Kelsey, G. & Constancia, M. Imprinted genes and the coordination of fetal and postnatal growth in mammals. *Novartis Foundation Symposia* **237** (2001), 19–42.

34. Chanoine, J. P., Yeung, L. P., Wong, A. C. & Birmingham, C. L. Immunoreactive ghrelin in human cord blood: relation to anthropometry, leptin, and growth hormone. *Journal of Pediatric Gastroenterology and Nutrition* **35** (2002), 282–286.

35. Bajoria, R., Sooranna, S. R., Ward, B. S. & Chatterjee, R. Prospective function of placental leptin at maternal-fetal interface. *Placenta* **23** (2002), 103–115.

36. Ehara, H., Ono, K. & Takeshita, K. Growth and development patterns in Prader–Willi syndrome. *Journal of Intellectual Disability Research* **37** (1993), 479–485.

Index